BEHAVIOR CHANGE IN THE CLASSROOM
Self-Management Interventions

The Guilford School Practitioner Series

EDITORS

STEPHEN N. ELLIOTT, Ph.D.
University of Wisconsin–Madison

JOSEPH C. WITT, Ph.D.
Louisiana State University, Baton Rouge

BEHAVIOR CHANGE IN THE CLASSROOM

Self-Management Interventions

EDWARD S. SHAPIRO, Ph.D.
CHRISTINE L. COLE, Ph.D.
Lehigh University

THE GUILFORD PRESS
New York   London

© 1994 The Guilford Press
A Division of Guilford Publications, Inc.
72 Spring Street, New York, NY 10012

Printed in the United States of America

This book is printed on acid-free paper.

Last digit is print number: 9   8   7   6   5   4   3   2   1

Library of Congress Cataloging-in-Publication Data

Shapiro, Edward S. (Edward Steven), 1951–
    Behavior change in the classroom : self-management interventions /
Edward S. Shapiro and Christine L. Cole.
        p.   cm. — (The Guilford school practitioner series)
    Includes bibliographical references (p.) and index.
    ISBN 0-89862-366-9
    1. Behavior modification. 2. Problem children—Education.
I. Cole, Christine L.   II. Title.   III. Series.
LB1060.2.S43   1994
370.15′3—dc20   93-42172
                                                                            CIP

*To my parents, who taught me to care
deeply about improving the lives of children
and the human condition (E.S.S.)*

For my parents, with love and gratitude (C.L.C.)

Preface

The goal of any behavior change process is to get individuals to display new, more adaptive patterns of behavior that will occur under the natural contingencies of every day experience. Such new behavior patterns will be long lasting, occur without reminders, and become a habitual part of the daily life of that individual. In a sense, this is what true learning is all about. Clearly, there would be no professional in the behavior change process who would dispute this claim.

If one sets this as the end product for an effective behavior change program, it should be clear that conceptualizing this process as the achievement of self-management makes sense. Indeed, self-management becomes the goal and expectation of every behavior change program we develop. This includes programs aimed at teaching new and more adaptive social and emotional responses as well as the learning of more academic tasks. Viewed this way, self-management suddenly becomes the goal of all teaching.

Despite the obvious importance of self-management in achieving behavior change, it is also important to note that there is a technology to achieving self-management that is not always understood or implemented by those who engage in behavior change strategies. Just like learning to ride a bike, throw a baseball, or read, self-management is a skill that must be learned. Although some level of self-management almost always occurs through maturation, it is also true that for children and youth who present with many academic, behavioral, and emotional difficulties, the level of self-management accomplished without specifically teaching these skills is far less than acceptable by others. Clearly, there is an important need for those who implement behavior change programs to have a strong knowledge of the technology of teaching self-management.

We have been engaged in research and training of self-management for much of our careers. I (E. S.) began exploring the use of self-management strategies with my doctoral dissertation. At that time, the research literature on self-management was in its infancy and my particular application, self-management of on-task behavior among young children with both moderate to severe mental retardation and severe emotional disturbance, had never been attempted. Since that successful study (Shapiro & Klein, 1979), I have examined the application of self-management strategies to children and adults with severely limited cognitive functioning levels, children with learning disabilities, and children with severe emotional disturbance. I have explored the application of self-management to academic skills such as spelling and math as well as vocational work skills.

My coauthor (C. C.), likewise, has been engaged in research and training in self-management throughout her professional life. She began her career applying self-management to adults with severe mental retardation as well as significant behavior problems. Her work has continued to examine how self-management can be applied to those with the most challenging behaviors in both school and nonschool settings. Most recently, she has shifted her efforts to applying the concept of self-management more broadly as choicemaking among youngsters with severe emotional disturbance.

Both of us strongly believe that the technology of self-management needs to be applied more consistently in school settings. Teachers, guidance counselors, school psychologists and other school personnel involved in working with children having behavioral difficulties need to understand how strategies to achieve self-management can be used in the routine aspects of teaching. This belief led to the current volume being written. The text was meant to provide a clear and practical guide for school-based professionals in how to put the techniques of teaching self-management into place in schools. Although appropriate rationale and research support for these techniques are included, the text more importantly emphasizes the practical considerations in using these strategies.

We sincerely hope the text accomplishes our goal of bringing the technology of self-management to the behavior change programs in schools. Although self-management, like any other process, is not a panacea for change, it certainly represents possibilities for more long-term, permanent behavior change processes. This must be the goal toward which we must strive.

As with any project like this, we would like to offer our sincere thanks to individuals who were instrumental in bringing this text to life. In particular, a special thanks is extended to Stephen N. Elliott who continues to be a driving force and inspiration in school psychology. His enthusiastic support and commitment to this text was certainly critical to its development. We would also like to thank Sharon Panulla, Senior Editor at The Guilford Press, who remains a strong supporter of this book and the entire School Practitioner series. We would also like to thank the many graduate students who have worked with us over the last several years and helped to produce the many case studies which are included in this text. Specifically, we would like to acknowledge the efforts of Christine Bankert, Jeanine Carfagno, Jennifer Pfannestiel, Cindy Ilgenfritz, and Dr. Elizabeth Pinter Lalli whose hard work at helping children we used as examples. The continued efforts of these and our many other students help us in maintaining the excitement and enthusiasm for our work.

Finally, we would like to offer our special thanks to our families. From me (Ed Shapiro), the love and support received from my wife Sally and two boys, Daniel and Jay, have allowed me to maintain my excitement for my work. While there certainly were times when they wanted me elsewhere, my family's understanding of my work is the centerpiece of our relationship that has always remained. From Chris Cole, special thanks to my husband, Jeff Kavanagh, for his good-natured support and understanding during this project, and to my daughters, Sarah and Megan, for being constant reminders of my priorities.

We hope that in some small way, this book will add to the betterment of the lives of troubled children and youth in school. That is the reason we continue to do what we do.

EDWARD S. SHAPIRO
CHRISTINE L. COLE
Lehigh University

Contents

1

Introduction

Most of the children in my classroom are making
satisfactory progress, but a few students are falling
behind academically and I've tried everything! They
just don't seem to have much initiative or
self-direction. How can I teach them to be more
motivated and independent?

I teach prevocational skills to adolescents with
severe disabilities. How can I be sure that the skills I
am teaching them here will transfer to their future
vocational settings?

There's a child in my second-grade class who is
extremely immature and anxious, especially in social
situations. I see the other students beginning to
reject her, and I'd like to do something to help her
become less anxious and more independent.

Some days my classroom is pure chaos! It seems all
I do is deal with one crisis after another. Is there
some way I could teach my students to get along
better and handle interpersonal conflicts on their
own so I'd have time to teach the things I want to
teach?

One of the primary goals of education is to ensure that children learn increasingly varied and complex skills of self-management. With these skills students may be able to complete a
task without teacher assistance, apply previously learned skills

in a new setting, become more self-assured, or resolve peer conflicts appropriately without adult intervention. As students develop skills of self-direction, they become less dependent on others to provide direction and incentive for their own behavior. Both students and teachers benefit directly from the shift away from exclusive teacher management of student behavior to increasing student self-management of their own actions.

Children with academic and behavior problems frequently have difficulty acquiring and using skills of self-management. In fact, one of the central features of many children with academic and behavior problems is an absence, or poorly-developed set, of self-management skills. These students typically have difficulty directing, controlling, inhibiting, or maintaining and generalizing behaviors needed for adaptive functioning in and outside the classroom.

Although the degree of self-management expected of students varies with age and ability level, some form of independence skills can be expected of even young children or children with severe disabilities. In fact, with the emphasis throughout the past decade on early intervention and normalization, there has been an increased interest in developing independence skills in at-risk preschoolers and persons with severe disabilities. In addition, children with mild or moderate mental retardation, learning disabilities, or serious emotional disturbance, must also develop skills of independence to ensure adaptive behavior functioning in and outside of school. Even many regular education students, who are often assumed to develop these skills automatically, could benefit from learning experiences designed to actively teach various self-management skills.

Although education personnel and parents alike agree that learning self-management skills is a priority for children, these skills are seldom systematically taught to students, especially those students with academic or behavior problems. The more typical emphasis has been on methods of classroom control and discipline using teacher-managed contingencies. Traditional behavior management or behavior modification strategies involving the external manipulation of antecedents and consequences have been successfully applied in response to a variety of discipline and instructional problems in school settings. Positive results using behavioral techniques have ranged from improving spelling accuracy (Stevens, Blackhurst, & Slaton, 1991) and increasing classroom participation (Narayan, Heward, Gardner, Courson, & Omness, 1990) to reducing serious problem behaviors (Charlop, Burgio, Iwata, & Ivancic, 1988). Token economies, differential reinforcement, and other positive reinforcement techniques have been used to increase desired classroom behaviors. Other procedures such as time out, response cost, and overcorrection have been shown to decrease undesired behaviors. Generally, these procedures are carried out on a daily basis by the teacher, who is also responsible for activities such as monitoring the child's progress and providing feedback to him or her.

LIMITATIONS OF TEACHER MANAGEMENT

Although these procedures have successfully remediated many types of classroom difficulties, practitioners have noted several limitations of traditional external management approaches. Ironically, students such as those with a serious emotional disturbance, who could benefit most from experiences designed to teach them skills for managing their own behavior, are frequently subjected to the tightest external management in an effort to "keep their behavior under control." This constant presence of strict external control typically does not allow these students the opportunities needed to learn how to manage their own actions. By limiting student involvement, as is frequently done in classrooms, we may be preventing students from developing those skills needed for them to become more self-reliant (Cole & Bambara, 1992).

There are several other potential limitations of external management strategies (Kazdin, 1975). Teachers may fail to notice many of a student's behaviors and thus provide consistent consequences for only a portion of his or her actions each day. As a result of this inconsistent responding, behavior change may be slow at best or, at worst, nonexistent. In addition, a teacher who administers the consequences for behavior may become a cue for the student's appropriate actions. As a result, appropriate behavior may occur only in the presence of the teacher. Student actions outside that particular teacher's purview may remain unchanged. Related to this, teachers may encounter difficulty promoting generalization of target behaviors to situations in which there are no externally-administered contingencies.

Another problem specifically associated with teacher-managed interventions to reduce disruptive behaviors in the classroom is that historically these have predominantly relied on punishment strategies. In fact, until recently, research investigations in this area were limited primarily to a study of how to best externally consequate behavior for most rapid suppression. Although potentially valuable in the short-term management of disruptive actions, external punishment procedures, when used as the major mode of intervention, do not actively teach students the skills necessary for long-term behavior change. And with the increased attention to the potential influence of teacher perceptions of interventions (Witt, 1986), additional limitations of these procedures have become apparent. For example, research indicates that teachers may hesitate to use particular interventions because they are perceived as being too behaviorally oriented, time demanding, or difficult to implement (Martens, Witt, Elliott, & Darveaux, 1985; Witt, Moe, Gutkin, & Andrews, 1984). These findings imply that an intervention strategy may be unsuccessful, not necessarily because the strategy itself is ineffective, but because it is not being used or is being used incorrectly (Martens & Meller, 1990). This would suggest a need for developing simple, cost-effective strategies with high utilization potential.

SELF-MANAGEMENT INTERVENTIONS

The drawbacks cited above, as well as other similar ethical, philosophical, and practical objections to the use of teacher-managed behavioral procedures, as well as an increased emphasis on the use of antecedent strategies for the prevention of student problems, have prompted the search for alternatives to these traditional approaches (Feldman & Peay, 1982; Strein, 1987). Recent emphasis has been on developing interventions designed to teach students specific skills of independence and self-reliance. One promising approach to enhancing independence and self-reliance in students with academic and behavioral difficulties is self-management interventions. Self-management interventions generally involve strategies related to changing or maintaining one's own behavior. Students are taught to use strategies that will increase appropriate academic or social behaviors and/or decrease inappropriate classroom behaviors. As such, self-management interventions address the philosophical and ethical concerns surrounding the use of external management by shifting responsibility for many of the intervention activities to the student, and by placing the primary focus on teaching children specific management or mediational skills.

Self-management strategies also appear to have high utilization potential (Fantuzzo & Polite, 1990). Many of the procedures are relatively easy to use and classroom demands on teachers may be reduced since students are taught to perform many of the time-consuming or routine classroom activities (e.g., monitoring, evaluating, graphing performance, delivering reinforcers). Finally, with the emphasis on teaching portable coping strategies that will transfer across behaviors and situations, self-management interventions have the potential for producing durable and generalizable behavior gains (see Holman & Baer, 1979; Whalen, Henker, & Hinshaw, 1985).

Interventions for teaching children to manage their own behavior in the classroom have burgeoned in the last two decades. Self-management interventions have been shown to effectively remediate a variety of academic and nonacademic problems exhibited by students of all ages and disability categories. Self-management interventions have been useful in such diverse areas as increasing homework completion in special education students in elementary schools (Fish & Mendola, 1986), increasing on-task behavior in students with learning disabilities (Hallahan, Marshall, & Lloyd, 1981), increasing reading workbook performance in students with behavior disorders (McLaughlin, Burgess, & Sackville-West, 1982), and decreasing disruptive behavior in children with hyperactivity (Christie, Hiss, & Lozanoff, 1984).

Defining Self-Management

Self-management generally refers to actions designed to change or maintain one's own behavior (Shapiro, 1981). Self-management interventions in the classroom involve teaching a child to engage in some behaviors (e.g., self-monitoring, self-instruction) in an effort to change a target behavior (e.g., completing math problems, talking out in class, paying attention). Although all self-management interventions assume that a child's problem behavior reflects a skill deficit, the broad umbrella of self-management encompasses a variety of approaches. These approaches vary from applied behavior analysis procedures emphasizing contingency management (e.g., Robertson, Simon, Pachman, & Drabman, 1979) to cognitive-behavioral approaches designed to teach children various mediational strategies (e.g., Kendall & Finch, 1978). Generally, *contingency-based* approaches target the consequences of behavior, whereas *cognitive-based* procedures focus more on the antecedents of behavior. The distinction between contingency-based and cognitive-based approaches is summarized in Table 1.1.

TABLE 1.1. Self-Management Interventions

Approaches	Focus	Examples of specific skills taught
Contingency-based	Consequences for appropriate and inappropriate behavior	Self-monitoring Self-evaluation Self-reinforcement
Cognitive-based	Antecedents for appropriate behavior	Self-instruction Stress-inoculation Social problem-solving

Contingency-Based Approaches

Typical skills associated with the contingency management approach include self-monitoring, self-evaluation, and self-reinforcement. With *self-monitoring*, children are instructed to observe specific aspects of their own behavior and provide an objective recording of these observations. Therefore, self-monitoring involves the two actions of self-observation and self-recording. Numerous studies have demonstrated that the activity of focusing attention on one's own behavior and the subsequent self-recording of these observations may result in positive reactive effects or improvement in the behavior being monitored (Gardner & Cole, 1988; Nelson, 1977; Shapiro & Cole, 1992). For example, Hughes and Hendrickson (1987) demonstrated the usefulness of self-monitoring with 12 fourth-, fifth-, and sixth-grade students, at risk for school maladjustment and academic failure. Students were taught to self-monitor their attention to a task at the sound of a tone, which was emitted on an average of every 30 seconds during independent seatwork. Results showed increased on-task behavior with these at-risk students following self-monitoring.

Self-evaluation involves the comparison of one's own behavior against a self-determined or externally-determined standard (Kanfer, 1977). For example, a teacher may have students rate their classroom behavior at the end of each period using a 5-point scale. Self-evaluation procedures have seldom been used alone and typically are included as one aspect of a multicomponent self-management package. For example, Smith, Young, West, Morgan, and Rhode (1988) evaluated the effectiveness of self-evaluation training taught within the context of a token program in reducing the disruptive and off-task behaviors of four junior high students in a special education resource classroom. Initially, students were informed of the classroom rules and rated their behavior on a scale of 0 to 5, according to how closely they followed these classroom rules. At the end of each class period, student ratings were compared with teacher ratings, with bonus points awarded for the matching of scores and a penalty imposed for failure to match. Points were exchangeable for snacks, school supplies, or magazines.

Matching requirements were gradually reduced and a simplified form of the procedure was introduced in the students' regular education classes. Results indicated that self-evaluation procedures implemented in the resource room reduced students' off-task and disruptive behaviors there, although little or no generalization of treatment gains were observed in the regular education classes.

As defined by Bandura (1976), *self-reinforcement* involves three conditions: (1) free access to reinforcers, (2) a self-imposed standard of performance that must be attained prior to reinforcement, and (3) self-determination that the performance criterion has been satisfied prior to reinforcement. While self-reinforcement procedures have appeared in some studies (typically as one component in a multicomponent package), they do not meet Bandura's criteria of independent self-reinforcement. Rather, self-reinforcement generally is limited to the act of self-delivering a consequence believed to have positive reinforcement qualities. For example, Pigott, Fantuzzo, Heggie, and Clement (1985) included self-reinforcement procedures in their evaluation of the effectiveness of student-administered procedures within a group context for increasing the arithmetic performance of four underachieving fifth-grade boys in a regular classroom. This intervention involved assigning a self-management role (i.e., self-instruction, self-observation, self-evaluation, and self-reinforcement) to each group member. The student responsible for self-evaluation and self-reinforcement activities (i.e., the "manager") performed such duties as adding up the team's score from the scorecard and comparing it with the team's goals for the day. If the goal was met, he declared the team had "won" and, after four wins, the group was eligible to obtain a group-determined back-up reinforcer. Results indicated that this group-oriented self-management program was effective in increasing the students' arithmetic performance to a point where it was indistinguishable from the performance of their classmates.

Cognitive-Based Approaches

Common cognitive-based approaches include *self-instruction training*, *stress inoculation training*, and *social problem-solving train-*

ing. Among the most popular of these is *self-instruction training*. As conceptualized by Meichenbaum (1977), the internalization of self-statements is important in the normal development of self-control behavior in children. Childhood behavior problems, in turn, are assumed to reflect deficient or maladaptive internalization of these self-statements (Dush, Hirt, & Schroeder, 1989). As a result, training in self-instruction involves teaching children specific verbalizations to direct their own behavior. In other words, it teaches them to talk to themselves. For example, the original Meichenbaum and Goodman (1971) study taught children with impulsive and hyperactive behavior to use overt, and eventually covert, speech to guide their overt actions. Since then, the efficacy of self-instruction approaches with children frequently has been demonstrated. For example, self-instruction training has been used effectively to increase academic behaviors such as on-task and independent work performance (Bornstein & Quevillon, 1976; Bryant & Budd, 1982) and academic accuracy (Roberts, Nelson, & Olson, 1987; Swanson & Scarpati, 1985), and to decrease disruptive behaviors (e.g., Burgio, Whitman, & Johnson, 1980; Kendall & Finch, 1978). However, self-instruction training has not always resulted in positive effects (e.g., Billings & Wasik, 1985; Friedling & O'Leary, 1979) and researchers have speculated that variables other than the self-instructions (i.e., good, clear instructions by another to perform the verbal and motor components of an activity, reinforcement for memorizing those instructions and reinforcement for accuracy in problem completion) may actually be responsible for the positive results obtained with this procedure (Roberts et al., 1987). Although questions such as these must be addressed by future investigations, the overall indication from the research to date is that self-instruction is a useful classroom procedure for some children.

Another cognitive-based self-management approach specifically designed to treat anger and anxiety problems in children is called *stress inoculation training*. This approach involves cognitive regulation and skills training for the management of anger or anxiety. The approach is based on the concepts of Lazarus (1976, 1977), who noted that cognitive processes play a central role in producing emotional arousal such as angry feelings. As a result, stress inoculation training is designed to develop a child's competence to adapt to stressful events. The term "inoculation" is a medical metaphor, which describes the central procedure of exposing the child to manageable doses of a stressor, thereby allowing him or her to gradually learn to cope. Examples include use of stress inoculation in group anger control training for junior high school dropouts (Feindler, Marriott, & Iwata, 1984), and to reduce anxiety over the transition to becoming a high school senior (Jason & Burrows, 1983).

A set of related cognitive-based procedures is referred to as *social problem-solving training*. The overall goal in social problem-solving approaches is to develop "thinking" skills that will enhance a student's social problem-solving behavior. Early work in this area suggested that aggressive or impulsive children exhibited deficits in generating alternative solutions to interpersonal problem situations (Spivack & Shure, 1974). Based on these findings, several different models of social problem solving were developed, all with the goal of enhancing these types of skills in order to remediate problem behaviors. The scope of social problem-solving training is generally more extensive than that of the other self-management interventions described. Social problem-solving approaches tend to be highly structured and include components such as problem identification, problem definition, generation of alternative solutions, evaluation of the consequences of alternative solutions, and implementation of the most appropriate solution (Keogh & Hall, 1984). A well-known example of the social problem-solving approach is the "Think Aloud" program, which involves teaching elementary-aged students to ask four basic questions when confronted with potentially difficult situations: "What is my problem?" "What is my plan?" "Am I using my plan?" and "How did I do?" (Camp, Blom, Hebert, & Van Doorninck, 1977).

One group of social problem-solving approaches is referred to as social skills training programs, which utilize many of the aspects of the other strategies previously described. Social skills training is based on an assumption that many behavior problems in children and adolescents (e.g., conduct disorders, depression, social isolation) are a result of specific social interactional skill deficiencies (Mash & Barkley, 1989). The primary objective of social skills training is to increase the student's ability to obtain reinforcement from others through more positive interpersonal interactions and, as a result, reduce the problem behavior(s). One of the most popular multifaceted social skills training programs is the Goldstein et al. (Goldstein, Sprafkin, Gershaw, & Klein, 1980; McGinnis & Goldstein, 1984) skill-streaming approach. With skill-streaming, students are taught a variety of skills to enhance social interactions, to use in planning, to deal with feelings, to replace aggressive responding, and to respond effectively to stress. Training is provided in a group format, typically with five to eight trainees, although it has also been implemented successfully in a regular-sized class within a school setting. The four components of each skill-streaming session are modeling, role playing, performance feedback, and transfer of training. Social skills training has been used successfully in school settings with children and adolescents who exhibit a range of problem behaviors.

SUMMARY

By now it is apparent that self-management interventions encompass a heterogeneous group of procedures, which have been used with children of all ages to remediate a wide variety of academic and behavior problems. Although heterogeneous, all of these strategies offer an alternative to traditional teacher-managed behavior modification approaches. With a focus on skill building, each of these self-management strategies attempts in some way to teach students to be more independent, self-reliant, and responsible for their own behavior.

The chapters in the present volume are organized with the education practitioner in mind. They provide detailed descriptions of the various self-management intervention strategies used in classroom settings. The techniques presented here are by no means exhaustive, but they do represent the most important self-management methods that have been applied in the treatment of academic and behavior problems in the schools. Chapter 2 provides examples from the empirical research literature of effective self-management interventions for academic and emotional/behavior problems in school settings. Major research findings are summarized and a discussion on generalization of self-management is provided. The next two chapters are devoted to specific intervention procedures. Chapter 3 provides practitioners with detailed descriptions and specific examples of how to implement contingency-based interventions. Chapter 4 provides, in similar detail, information and specific examples of how to implement cognitive-based interventions in the classroom. In these chapters, both academic and behavior problems are targeted and practical suggestions for implementation of each intervention are provided. Chapter 5 describes how self-management strategies can be applied to students with severe disabilities. Additional general implementation issues likely to be encountered in using self-management with all students are addressed in more detail in Chapter 6. Finally, Chapter 7 describes several cases demonstrating how problems identified in the classroom can be dealt with successfully using self-management interventions. It is our hope that the information in this volume is provided in sufficient detail to allow interested readers to design and implement their own self-management interventions with children and adolescents in school settings.

2

Review of the Literature

Over the last decade, a substantial literature has emerged delineating the use of self-management techniques. These procedures have been applied across individuals in regular classrooms, as well as across those with a wide range of identified handicapping conditions such as severe mental retardation (Shapiro, Browder, & D'Huyvetters, 1984), moderate and mild levels of mental retardation (Hughes, Korineck, & Gorman, 1991), learning disabilities (e.g., Hallahan et al., 1981), and serious emotional disturbance (Nelson, Smith, Young, & Dodd, 1991). Self-management has also been applied across a wide variety of academic problems including homework completion (Fish & Mendola, 1986), on-task behavior (e.g., Hallahan et al., 1981), reading performance (McLaughlin et al., 1982), and math computation (Skinner, Turco, Beatty, & Rasavage, 1989). Applications across nonacademic problems have also been widespread including such targets as hyperactive behavior (Christie et al., 1984), task productivity in a workshop environment (Shapiro & Ackerman, 1983), and social problem-solving skills (Shapiro, 1989). Researchers have examined how individual components of self-management can impact behavior change (DiGangi, Maag, & Rutherford, 1991), as well as how multicomponent packages effect change (Brigham, 1989). Additional research has provided insights into how self-management can be potentially used for purposes of achieving generalization and maintenance after behavior change has been accomplished through teacher-managed behavioral interventions (e.g., Rhode, Morgan, & Young, 1983). Finally, other investigators have written about the conceptual underpinnings of self-management processes (e.g., Mace & Kratochwill, 1985; Mace & West, 1986). With little question, there is an extensive knowledge base, which has developed in a very short period.

Obviously, it would be virtually impossible to provide an extensive and exhaustive review of this literature in the space allotted for this book. Interested readers are encouraged to examine the numerous reviews of the literature that have appeared over the last several years, which summarize much of the self-management research. A list of these reviews and their focus is provided in Table 2.1. In this chapter, a brief review of studies that have employed self-management for school-based problems is presented, which is divided into two major subsections: one examining self-management for attentional and academic skills problems, and the other focusing on its application to nonacademic problems.

ATTENTIONAL AND ACADEMIC SKILLS PROBLEMS

Attentional Difficulties

A substantial number of studies have focused on the improvement of attention or on-task behavior as the variable of interest. Indeed, many of the earliest studies on classroom self-management examined how procedures such as self-monitoring or self-recording could effectively improve a child's attention to tasks (e.g., Glynn & Thomas, 1974; Broden, Hall, & Mitts, 1971). Hallahan et al. (1981) provided a good example of the procedures used in most of these studies. In their study, three 10-year-old students, classified as learning disabled, were found to have low levels of attention to their work during a 45-minute reading comprehension lesson. Following baseline data collection, students were given wrist counters. A tape recording was developed that played audible beeps between 10

TABLE 2.1. Review Articles on Self-Management and Their Focus

Authors and year of publication	Focus of Review
Fantuzzo & Polite (1990)	Analyzed school-based interventions with elementary school students.
Fantuzzo, Polite, Cook, & Quinn (1988)	Compared teacher- vs. student-managed classroom interventions for children
Fantuzzo, Rohrbeck, & Azar (1987)	Conducted a component analysis of school-based self-management interventions.
Fox & Kendal (1983)	Reviewed self-instruction training for improving academic skill problems
Grossman & Hughes (1992)	Perfomed meta-analyses of self-management for students with internalizing disorders.
Hughes, Korinek, & Gorman (1991)	Analyzed public-school-based interventions for students with mental retardation.
Hughes, Ruhl, & Misra (1989)	Researched public-school-based interventions for students formally identified as having a behavior disorder or similar label (e.g., emotionally disturbed, emotionally handicapped).
Nelson, Smith, Young, & Dodd (1991)	Reviewed classroom-based interventions with students identified as having a behavior disorder or similar classification (e.g., hyperactive, socially maladjusted).
Roberts & Dick (1982)	Analyzed classroom-based interventions, comparing contigency-managed and cognitive-change approaches to self-management.

and 90 seconds apart. These tones were set to occur on average every 45 seconds. Students were instructed to ask themselves the question "Was I paying attention?" at the sound of each tone. Over a 3-day period, students were trained in the application of the procedure. In particular, students needed to demonstrate accurate discrimination of the presence or absence of their on-task behavior at the sound of the tone.

Results of the study showed increases in on-task behavior across all three students from initial levels of 20–30% of the observed intervals to 50–80%. After successful implementation for about 20 days, both the wrist counter and tape recorder were faded with on-task behavior maintaining its level present before fading began.

Other studies have used very similar self-monitoring approaches when trying to improve on-task behavior. Employing the same procedures, Hallahan, Lloyd, Kneedler, and Marshall (1982) compared the use of self-monitoring to teacher-monitoring of on-task behavior in an 8-year-old student with learning disabilities. Results again showed good improvement over baseline levels of 40% on-task to over 90% on-task for both types of monitoring. In addition, Hallahan et al. (1982) found the self-monitoring condition to result in somewhat higher performance than teacher monitoring.

Hughes and Hendrickson (1987) used the procedure described by Hallahan et al. (1981) to improve the on-task behavior of 12 fourth-, fifth-, and sixth-grade students in a regular education classroom, who were selected because they were considered at risk for academic failure. Again, an audible tone was played at random intervals ranging from 15 to 90 seconds, averaging every 30 seconds. Students were trained to ask themselves, "Was I paying attention when the tone went off?" Students were instructed to record their answer by checking a box ("Yes" or "No") on a recording form attached to their desk.

Results of the study were consistent with the findings of Hallahan's studies. Again, the self-monitoring of on-task behavior increased the students' attentiveness from initial levels of around 50–60% of the observed intervals to over 80% for most students. There was some variability among the students, with two showing little change between the baseline and intervention phases.

Prater, Joy, Chilman, Temple, and Miller (1991) used this procedure with adolescents with learning disabilities. Students in their study ranged in age from 12 years, 11 months to 17 years, 2 months. Across the five students, the self-monitoring procedure was implemented in a resource room for math, a self-contained special education classroom, a study hall for social studies, and a resource room for government and English. In addition, instead of training students to simply ask themselves if they were paying attention, Prater et al. (1991) used a visual prompter (a sign displayed in the front of the room) to assist students in remembering to self-monitor. Audio tones were played using random intervals ranging from 1 to 2.5 minutes. For all students, use of the audio tone cues were faded as well as use of the self-monitoring recording sheet.

Results of the study showed consistent and strong effects across all students. Following baseline, on-task behavior showed dramatic and immediate improvements. Baseline levels varied across students but averaged around 40% of observed intervals. Improvements to over 80% were noted across students.

It is particularly important to note that the dramatic effects of these studies resulted from a relatively simple intervention. In each case, students were taught how to self-monitor their on-task behavior and did so whenever an audible tone was played. For many students, no additional externally provided reinforcement was necessary. The process of self-monitoring was reactive and resulted in substantial improvements in the targeted behavior. While such effects are not always as dramatic as these nor maintained over time (e.g., Shapiro et al., 1984; Shapiro, McGonigle, & Ollendick, 1981), and such changes can be very idiosyncratic (Shapiro et al., 1984), it is clear that the self-monitoring of on-task behavior can have a significant impact on many students.

Academic Skills Problems

A number of studies have applied self-management procedures specifically to academic skills problems. Although some of these studies have employed procedures similar to those used for monitoring on-task behavior, others have used more complex multicomponent self-management procedures. In addition, while the self-monitoring of on-task behavior tends to be implemented using a contingency management approach to self-management, procedures developed for academic skills problems have involved both contingency-based and cognitive-based techniques.

Contingency-Based Procedures

Piersel (1985) reported a study in which a self-monitoring procedure was used with an 8-year-old third-grade boy who had a significant problem with work completion. Prior to implementing the procedure, this boy had never completed more than 40% of his assigned daily independent work. The intervention procedure required the child to record the completion of assignments as he handed them to the teacher. The chart was then checked during weekly meetings between the child and a psychologist. Recorded on the child's chart were assignment completions across the entire day, including reading, spelling, penmanship, language, mathematics, science, and health. An assignment had to be 80% accurate to be considered complete. Total number of assignments per day ranged from four to nine.

Results were dramatic and immediate. As soon as the procedure was implemented, the child completed 75–100% of all assignments. This was maintained through a phase during which the weekly meetings were discontinued. A particularly important aspect of this procedure was the absence of additional rewards beyond those normally provided to the students in the classroom for completing his assignment (i.e., less homework, fewer teacher-directed reprimands, fewer incomplete assignment notices to parents).

Szykula, Saudargas, and Wahler (1981) reported a study in which two fifth-grade students were taught to self-record the number of math problems assigned, the number completed, and the number correct during an arithmetic class. In addition, the use of goal setting as well as contingent rewards were added to the self-recording task during subsequent phases. Results of their study showed somewhat different effects for each of the two boys. For one boy, little change in behavior was evident until contingent rewards were added to the package. For the other student, the addition of the goal-setting procedure appeared to be the key component.

An important finding of this study, which reinforces those of other studies, is that the effects of self-monitoring are idiosyncratic in nature. While in previous studies self-monitoring alone was shown to result in substantial changes in student performance, neither child in this study showed reactive responses to self-monitoring. Instead, procedures added to the self-monitoring condition were necessary to achieve improved behavior. Indeed, for one child, two procedures (goal setting and contingent reward) were needed before change became evident. Of course, it is also possible that for either child the use of goal setting or contingent reward alone may have been equally as effective as those procedures combined with self-monitoring.

Lalli and Shapiro (1990) reported a study that specifically targeted the use of self-monitoring in the acquisition of "sight" words for students with learning disabilities. A total of eight students (first through sixth grades) enrolled in a self-contained private school for students with learning disabilities participated. All students were on average 2.1 years behind their same-age peers in reading. During prebaseline assessment, a series of word lists were constructed from the students' reading material. These lists included a pool of 75 unknown vocabulary words, divided into five lists of 15 words each. An attempt was made to equate the lists for words with similar length.

The intervention procedure involved having students read their word list while a tape recording of the words being read was played at 5-second intervals. After students read each word and then heard it read correctly on their tape recordings, they were instructed to mark either a "+" or "−" to indicate if they had read the word correctly. Students were trained to record a "+" only if they finished reading the word before the tape-recorded version of the word was heard. Once a list was mastered (12 of 15 words recorded accurately on two consecutive sessions), a new list was introduced for the next phase.

Lalli and Shapiro (1990) examined the differential effects of self-monitoring alone versus self-monitoring combined with contingent rewards. Results, displayed in Figure 2.1, showed that the self-monitoring condition resulted in almost equal performance across students compared to when a contingent reward was added to self-monitoring. More importantly for this discussion, the use of self-monitoring for acquiring "sight" word vocabulary among students with learning disabilities was successful.

Several other studies illustrate how self-management techniques can be applied directly for improving specific aca-

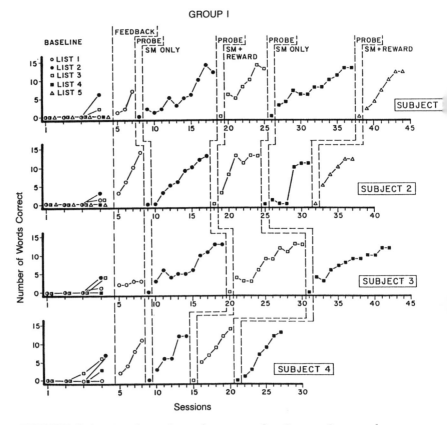

FIGURE 2.1. Number of words correct for Group One students. From *The Effects of Self-Monitoring and Contingent Reward on Sight Word Acquisition* (p. 136) by E. P. Lalli and E. S. Shapiro, 1990, Pittsburgh: Pressley Ridge School. Copyright 1990 by Pressly Ridge School. Reprinted by permission.

demic skills problems. For example, Stowitschek, Ghezzi, and Safely (1987) examined the use of self-evaluation and self-correction procedures in improving the letter formation of students classified as mildly mentally retarded. In the first of a series of two studies, Stowitschek et al. (1987) identified four students (ages 10 to 13) from a classroom who copied fewer than three letters of the alphabet correctly. Using correction templates, students were taught to self-evaluate their performance on daily writing assignments. Following an eight-step procedure, students were instructed to (1) complete the first row of the daily worksheet, (2) place the template under the worksheet, (3) align the template with the worksheet, (4) highlight missed letters with a transparent felt tip marker, (5) remove the template, (6) erase incorrect portions of highlighted letters, (7) correct the highlighted letters with a pencil, and (8) move to the next row completing only those letters that needed to be corrected from the previous row. This procedure was taught through modeling until students demonstrated that they could do it independently. The procedure was learned across 3 days by all four students.

Results were dramatic. All four students showed substantial improvements in the number of letters formed correctly. From baselines of near zero, students improved through intervention and follow-up reinforcement to completing four to six letters correctly per session. All four students were able to learn to use the procedure, taking between 22 and 40 sessions to attain criterion performance across all eight steps on the initial worksheet. On subsequent worksheets, students showed significantly improved performance, reaching criterion levels in almost one-half as many sessions. In a follow-up study, Stowitschek et al. (1987) taught regular classroom teachers to implement the procedures with a new set of students. The results of this study replicated the outcomes of the first study.

Dunlap and Dunlap (1989) reported the results of a study in which three students with learning disabilities used a self-monitoring procedure to assist them in mastering subtraction. Following a two-phase baseline during which students were given verbal instructions on how to perform subtraction problems as well as points for successful academic performance that were already part of the regular classroom management system, a self-monitoring package was taught. Based on an error analysis of each student's performance during baseline, individualized checklists were developed. Checklists were constructed so that the list of items students were trained to self-monitor represented the types of errors they typically made. For example, for one student the checklist included the following items:

1. I copied the problem correctly.
2. I regrouped when I needed to (top number is bigger than bottom number).
3. I borrowed correctly (number crossed out is one bigger).
4. I subtracted all the numbers.
5. I subtracted correctly.

For another student the list consisted of these items:

1. I underlined all the top numbers that were smaller than the bottom ones.
2. I crossed out only the number next to the underlined number and made it one less.
3. I put a "1" beside the underlined number.
4. All the numbers on the top are bigger than the numbers on the bottom.

During the self-monitoring phase, students were expected to place a "+" or "−" next to each item on the checklist, which corresponded to a particular problem. If a minus sign was recorded, the student reworked the problem without erasing the original attempt. Students were awarded points for correct responses and additional points for each problem in which all steps on the self-monitoring checklist were correctly recorded. A maintenance phase was implemented after students had established and maintained high levels of self-monitored responding. Findings showed that self-monitoring resulted in the performance of better than 75% of items correct for all students. These levels of performance were maintained when the self-monitoring checklists were removed.

Kapadia and Fantuzzo (1988) compared the relative effects of a teacher-managed versus a self-management procedure to improve spelling performance among four students with learning disabilities. During a daily spelling drill activity, students were either assessed and reinforced by the teacher for their performance or engaged in self-monitoring and self-reinforcement. Results showed clearly that students performed better under the self-management condition.

In a somewhat more comprehensive package using self-evaluation for behavior change, Glomb and West (1990) described the use of a procedure they called "WATCH" in targeting assignment completion, grammatical accuracy, and neatness of penmanship among two high school students classified as behavior disordered. Using creative writing assignments as the targeted task, data were collected on the completeness, grammatical accuracy, and neatness of weekly writing activities. Following baseline, students were trained to use self-instruction and self-questioning activities to implement the various parts of the "WATCH" intervention. This included: *W*riting down assignments and their due dates; *A*sking for clarification or help if needed; *T*ask-analyzing the assignment and scheduling the tasks over the days available to complete the assignment; and *CH*ecking all work for completeness, accuracy, and neatness. During the training, students were asked to rate themselves using a point system on how well they had adhered to the strategy and met the preset criteria set by the teacher. Similar ratings were made by the teacher. Exact matches were rewarded with bonus points, matches within one point resulted in students being awarded the number of points they themselves determined that they deserved, and differences of more than one point resulted in students not receiving any points.

Results of the study showed substantial improvements in the percentage of words completed on writing assignments from initial near-zero levels to between 70% and 100% of the words correct on weekly assignments. These results again showed the particularly powerful effects that self-evaluation, goal setting, and self-regulation can play in improving as complex a skill as creative writing.

Cognitive-Based Procedures

A substantial number of studies have been conducted in which self-instruction training or some derivative of self-instruction training has been used to improve academic skills. In general, self-instruction training is a technique originally reported by Meichenbaum and Goodman (1971), where students are taught to talk out loud as they engage in problem solving. Several studies illustrative of the range of studies reported in the literature are presented. Interested readers should examine some of the review articles noted in Table 2.1 for more detail.

Burgio et al. (1980) reported an investigation involving two students, 9 and 11 years old, identified as having mild levels of mental retardation, who had difficulties in task completion in the areas of math and penmanship. An extensive training program was implemented outside the classroom during which the students were taught to model the use of talking out loud to themselves as they solved each problem. After the training was completed, it was found that the students applied the self-instruction technique during the math and penmanship activities in the classroom setting. Results of the study showed that the students decreased their levels of off-task behavior significantly as a function of using the self-instruction training program, although little change in performance on the academic task was found. However, this was not a primary objective of the study; the self-instructions were primarily aimed at improving on-task behavior rather than the academic skill itself.

In a follow-up study, however, Johnston, Whitman, and Johnson (1980) employed a self-instruction sequence that was specifically designed to teach students with mild mental retardation to perform addition and subtraction using regrouping. An example of the script used for self-instruction for developing addition is provided in Table 2.2. Results of their study showed that students demonstrated substantial increases

TABLE 2.2. Example of Self-Instruction Training Sequence for Addition with Regrouping

Q. What kind of a problem is this?

$$\begin{array}{r} 36 \\ +47 \\ \hline \end{array}$$

A. It's an add problem, I can tell by the sign.

Q. Now what do I do?

A. I start with the top numer in the one's column and I add. Six and 7 (the child points to the 6 on a number line and counts down 7 spaces) is 13. Thirteen has two digits. That means I have to carry. This is hard so I go slowly. I put the 3 in the one's column (the child writes the 3 in the one's column) and the 1 in the ten's column (the child writes the 1 above the top number in the ten's column).

Q. Now what do I do?

A. I start with the top number in the ten's column. One add 3 (the child points to the 1 on the number line and counts down 3 spaces) is 4. Four add 4 (the child counts down 4 more spaces) is 8 (the child writes the 8 in the ten's column).

Q. I want to get it right so I check it. How do I check it?

A. I cover up my answer (the child covers the answer with a small piece of paper) and add again starting with the bottom number in the one's column. Seven add 6 (the child points to the 7 on the number line and counts down 6 spaces) is 13 (the child slides the piece of paper to the left and uncovers the 3; he or she sees the 1 which he/she has written over the top number in the ten's column. Got it right. Four add 3 (the child points to the 4 on the number line and counts down 3 spaces) is 7. Seven add 1 (the child counts down 1 more space) is 8 (the child removes the small piece of paper so that the entire answer is visible). I got it right so I'm doing well. (If, by checking his or her work, the child determines that he or she has made an error, he or she says, "I got it wrong. I can fix it if I go slowly." The child then repeats the self-instruction sequence starting from the beginning.)

Note. Adapted from "Teaching Addition and Subtraction to Mentally Retarded Children: A Self-Instruction Program by M. B. Johnston, T. L. Whitman, and M. Johnson, 1980, *Applied Research in Mental Retardation, 1,* p. 149. Copyright 1980 by Pergamon Press. Reprinted by permission.

in academic performance related to the implementation of the self-instruction program for addition and subtraction skills. A particularly interesting aspect of their study was that students did not automatically apply the self-instruction technique learned first for addition to the subtraction activities. Instead, students had to be prompted through the self-instruction sequence for subtraction before they would begin using the technique with that activity. Whitman and Johnston (1983) provided similar outcomes in a replication of this study. This suggests that generalization of self-instruction skills to untrained tasks may not occur automatically and that trainers may need to actively teach self-instruction in each targeted academic subject.

Fish and Mendola (1986) reported a study that examined the effectiveness of self-instruction training in improving homework assignment completion rates for three children identified as emotionally disturbed. Self-instruction training was provided using the Meichenbaum and Goodman (1971) technique across tasks in mathematics, reading, and language arts. In this procedure, self-instructions are initially modeled by the trainer by talking out loud. Over time, the student learns to talk to themselves without the trainer's help. The specific self-instructions were designed around homework completion. An example of the trainer's model would be: "Now what time is it? Oh! Time for me to do my homework. Where am I going to do it? I know, I'll do it in the _____ (whatever room subject usually does homework in). Now, what homework do I have for tonight? Okay, first I'll do _____ then _____ and then _____. Good! It looks like I have a lot to do, but I'll do the best I can. If my mind wanders, I'll tell myself, 'Back to work!' After I'm finished, I can play" (Fish & Mendola, 1986, p. 270). Students were trained individually for eight 30-minute sessions over a 2-week period.

Results of the study showed that all students had substantial improvements in their rates of homework completion after the implementation of the self-instruction training. These ranged from approximately 25% of assignments completed in baseline to 75–100% of assignments completed after training was completed. A remarkable outcome of this study was that the self-instruction training, conducted outside of the regular classroom environment and not centered on any particular type of assignment alone, resulted in improved homework completion across different types of tasks. Although there are some questions about the degree to which the self-instruction training per se was responsible for the change in assignment completion rate, the study did illustrate the potential power of such a technique to influence change in student behavior.

Miller, Miller, Wheeler, and Selinger (1989) examined the use of self-instruction techniques to improve the academic performance of two boys, 11 and 12 years old, currently enrolled in an institutional setting for students with emotional disturbance. With the first boy, a procedure known as "touch-math" was taught using self-instruction techniques. This procedure involved teaching the student to look at the top number in a subtraction problem, regroup if needed, place the corresponding number of dots on the numbers in the subtrahend, say the top number, and count backwards to obtain the answer. Once the answer was reached, the student was taught to verbalize the entire subtraction process and then check his answer by reversing the process. Using the typical sequence of modeling and faded prompts described by Meichenbaum and Goodman (1971), the student was taught this procedure over a 4-day period. Following somewhat erratic performance after the initial intervention, additional self-monitoring procedures were added in which a checklist was generated to assist the student in performing the necessary self-instructional steps.

For the second student, a self-instruction procedure designed to assist the student in decoding words was developed. The three steps of the self-instruction technique consisted of the following: (1) Ask yourself, "What is the sound of the first letter?", (2) then ask, "Does it look like another word that I do know?", and (3) finally blank out the letter and read the rest of the sentence. Again, this technique was taught to the student using a shortened version of the Meichenbaum and Goodman (1971) procedure.

Results for both boys were impressive with the self-instruction procedure. They showed improvements from consistently zero correct for the first child in baseline, to 90–100% correct through the intervention period. Results for the second student were not quite as dramatic, but nevertheless showed improvements from 60–70% in baseline to 80–90% during the intervention period. In both cases, these levels of performance were maintained as the self-instruction program was faded.

Esposito, Cole, Shapiro, and Bambara (1993) describe a cognitive-based procedure for improving the study skills of high school biology students in a regular education classroom. In their study, Esposito developed a four-step intervention program, which included self-scoring, self-graphing, question/answer generation, and oral summarization. Using a classwide implementation across 19 students enrolled in a regular tenth grade biology class, the self-scoring phase of the intervention was first begun. Using the scores on daily quizzes, a total of 4 students met the preestablished criteria and did not need implementation of any additional parts of the intervention package. Self-graphing was added to self-scoring for the remaining 15 students in the class. This resulted in 4 additional students meeting criterion. The third component, developing questions from assigned homework and writing answers to these questions, was then implemented with the remaining 11 students, resulting in 6 more students meeting criterion. Only the 5 students who had not responded to the use of the previous intervention components were trained to engage in all four of the self-management components.

Results of the Esposito et al. (1993) study suggest that self-management procedures that are employed with homework activities can be very powerful methods for improving the study skills of high school students in a content area class such as biology. More importantly, this study also showed that it may be unnecessary to implement all components of a self-management system for all students. Indeed, only 5 of 19 students really required the complete cognitive-behavioral self-management package before their quiz grades reached preset criterion levels.

Among the many self-management procedures that have been developed for improving academic skills problems using cognitive-based procedures such as self-instruction, those developed by applied researchers at the University of Kansas Institute for Research in Learning Disabilities have had perhaps the most significant impact. Since 1977, this group has been engaged in developing techniques aimed at improving the academic skill performance of middle and secondary school students with learning disabilities. In particular, their efforts have focused on developing strategies for learning that can be applied broadly across content area instruction. All of their work has emphasized the need for self-managed learning (see Lenz, 1992, for a review and discussion of much of this work).

Entitled the Strategies Intervention Model (Deshler & Schumaker, 1988), the major objective of this work was to teach students how to regulate their own academic performance in an independent and interdependent way. The focus has consistently been on teaching students to engage in cognitive regulation and to combine various strategies into an integrated package that will enhance student performance across different academic subjects.

Research on the use of self-managed strategies has been extensive. In general, it has focused on four strands—the acquisition, storage, expression, and demonstration of knowledge in a subject area through tests and assignments. In each of these domains, students are taught certain strategies as well as a means to integrate these strategies across and within domains. Table 2.3 illustrates the many different strategies that have been developed in each domain.

Learning strategies that researchers have developed fall into roughly four categories: (1) those focused on teaching students to acquire information, (2) those focused on helping students store information, (3) those used to aid them in expressing information in writing, and (4) those focusing on the ability to demonstrate competence on tests and assignments. Each strategy has undergone extensive field testing and ongoing evaluation. A substantial research base exists in the literature reporting the outcomes for each of these strategies.

One of the acquisition strategies developed is called multipass. The purpose of this strategy is to teach students how to

TABLE 2.3. Strategy Systems Based on the Strategies Intervention Model

Strategy systems	Skills that are taught
Acquisition strategies	
Word identification	Identify unfamiliar words in text
Paraphrasing reading	Paraphrase text to improve comprehension
Self-questioning	Ask and answer questions while reading
Visual-imagery	Visualize settings and action during reading
Interpreting visuals	Inspect visuals in text for information
Multipass	Read a chapter of text for key information
Storage strategies	
FIRST-letter mnemonic	Organize and remember lists of information
Paired associates	Remember pairs or small groups of information
Listening and notetaking	Listen for, note, and organize information
Expression strategies	
Sentence writing	Write simple/compound/complex sentences
Paragraph writing	Write basic and complex paragraphs
Error monitoring	Identify and correct writing errors
Theme writing	Write five creative paragraphs on a theme
Demonstration of competence strategies	
Test taking	Approach tests effectively and efficiently
Assignment completion	Complete assignments more effectively

Note. Adapted from "Self-managed Learning Strategy Systems for Children and Youth" by B. Keith Lenz, 1992, *School Psychology Review, 21,* p. 214. Copyright 1992 by the National Association of School Psychologists. Reprinted by permission.

access information from a textbook chapter by repeatedly going over the chapter. On each pass through, students are taught to look for and acquire specific types of information. Schumaker, Deshler, Alley, Warner, and Denton (1982) examined the use of this strategy among eight high school students with learning disabilities. Their research demonstrated that students could be taught the use of the complex multipass strategy and that this use resulted in the significantly improved acquisition of information from a textbook chapter. They further found that students could apply the strategy in both easy- and grade-level textbooks and, as a result, scored better on tests taken in their regular classrooms. Lenz (1992) noted that while multipass was being developed, it was found that some students were unable to learn the strategy because they lacked specific text-processing strategies. This resulted in the development of specific acquisition strategies such as those listed in Table 2.2.

Storage strategies focus on teaching students how to store information for future use. One such strategy, the "FIRST-letter mnemonic" strategy, was designed to teach students a method for organizing information into lists and developing mnemonic strategies for remembering their contents (Nagel, Schumaker, & Deshler, 1986). Research on this strategy has shown that students perform substantially better on regular classroom exams after learning to use it.

Expression strategies have focused on written expression by teaching students how to write and check their work. Included are sentence writing, paragraph writing, error monitoring, and theme writing strategies. Again, studies conducted on these strategies have shown very positive outcomes among high school students with learning disabilities (e.g., Schumaker, Deshler, Alley, Warner, Clark, & Nolan, 1982).

Procedures Designed to Improve Attentional and Academic Skills

Over the last decade, several researchers have tried to examine the interrelationships between targeting on-task behaviors versus academic skills problems. Klein (1979), in a thorough review of earlier research, concluded that studies that targeted on-task behavior may result in improvements in attentional behavior, but were unlikely to show consistent change in academic performance. In contrast, studies that focused on academic performance were able to show consistent improvements in on-task behavior. Based upon his review, Klein made clear recommendations that applied researchers consider targeting academic performance even when on-task behavior appears to be the primary referral problem. Similar findings and recommendations were echoed by Snider (1987).

Several researchers have continued to examine this important collateral relationship between on-task behavior and academic performance. McLaughlin (1983) reported a study in which a self-monitoring procedure for on-task behavior was implemented for three 8- to 9-year-old boys in a classroom for students with behavior disorders. In his study, students were given a sheet of paper marked with squares and were told to make a "+" whenever they felt they were studying (an example of on-task behavior) and a "−" when they were not. No cueing device or other prompt to self-monitor was employed. Students were told to simply self-monitor when they remembered to do so. Data were obtained on both the students' on-task behavior and the percent correct on daily assignments in handwriting, spelling, and math. Results showed that all students improved their on-task behavior substantially over baseline levels. Similarly, overall improvements in accuracy of academic performance were noted. McLaughlin notes that others have also found similar improvements in academic performance when only on-task behavior is targeted (Hallahan et al., 1981, 1982; McLaughlin, 1984; McLaughlin & Truhlicka, 1983).

Hughes and Boyle (1991) examined the interrelationship between self-monitoring on-task behavior and academic performance among three students with moderate retardation. In this study, the rates of accurate task completion across seven different types of tasks were examined. Self-monitoring using the same type of technique described above by Hallahan et al. (1981) was used. Results showed that levels of task completion for two of the three students improved substantially when on-task behavior was monitored. For one student, however, only on-task behavior showed increases. Performance on the tasks remained stable or showed slight increases not directly related to improvements in on-task behavior.

In an attempt to provide a more definitive answer to the question of the relationship between on-task behavior and academic task productivity, Lloyd, Bateman, Landrum, and Hallahan (1989) had five students identified as either seriously emotionally disturbed or learning disabled engage in either self-monitoring of on-task behavior or academic productivity. In both conditions, correct academic performance and on-task behavior were simultaneously measured.

Results showed that neither procedure produced clearly differential effects for academic productivity or on-task behavior. Both procedures resulted in substantially higher performance than baseline. When students were asked to indicate their choice of procedures, they elected to self-monitor on-task behavior rather than academic performance. During these phases, on-task behavior and academic productivity remained at levels equivalent to previous phases.

In a similar type of study, Harris (1986) examined the effects of having four children identified as learning disabled self-monitor their on-task behavior or their degree of academic productivity during a spelling lesson. Following baseline, self-monitoring procedures previously described by Hallahan et al. (1981), which aimed at increasing on-task behavior, were implemented for two students, while the other two students self-monitored their academic productivity. After 10 school days, self-monitoring of the opposite behavior was instituted.

Results showed that on-task behavior increased over baseline during all treatment phases. Changes to academic productivity rates were evident when self-monitoring was used for either behavior, although superior results were noted for one subject when academic productivity was monitored rather than on-task behavior. Results for the other students were less clear.

Lam, Cole, Shapiro, and Bambara (in press) examined the interrelationships of on-task behavior, academic productivity, and disruptive behavior among students with serious emotional disturbance. In this study, students were taught to self-monitor each of these problem behaviors, and engaged in the self-monitoring during different phases of the study. In each phase, data were collected on the collateral responses.

Results of their study showed that the behavior that was

being directly self-monitored tended to show the most desirable outcomes. Among the three behaviors, the self-monitoring of academic accuracy tended to produce the most consistent collateral effects on on-task and disruptive behaviors.

Overall, the original recommendation of Klein (1979) and Snider (1987) that self-monitoring should focus on academic responses rather than on-task behavior does not seem totally justified. There have been enough contrasting research findings to suggest that monitoring on-task behavior, an easier procedure than monitoring academic responses, should be considered a viable alternative for producing behavior change. Indeed, for many students, the monitoring of on-task behavior may result in increased academic productivity. Although one would certainly predict that the monitoring of academic responses would almost always result in improved on-task behavior, its limited acceptance by many students (e.g., Lloyd et al., 1989) may make it less attractive as an initial intervention plan. Similarly, it is important to note that the jury is still out on this question. Clearly, the contrasting research findings may be due to many uncontrolled and unexplained variables such as how academic productivity is measured, the age of the students, the particular type of handicapping condition the students have, the nature of the task, and so forth. Continued efforts to clearly resolve this question are needed.

Conclusions and Summary

From this brief review of the self-management literature, it should be clear that these procedures can play a major role in the development of effective interventions for behavior change among students. They are widely applicable across various types of problems, ages of students, academic tasks, content areas, areas of basic instruction, and cognitive abilities. More importantly, they provide a somewhat simple but extremely important means for enhancing the self-regulation that all teachers seek to achieve in students. Many of the techniques are not difficult to implement nor are they difficult to monitor. Yet, they offer to practitioners proven methods for affecting

long-term and potentially permanent change in student behavior.

Despite the proliferation of research in self-management
for academic skills problems, many questions remain. For example, the exact longevity of changes resulting from these
interventions is unknown. While it is believed that such interventions implemented over a long-term period should result
in maintenance of behavior change in students, few, if any,
longitudinal examinations of self-management processes have
been reported in the literature.

Another important question about these procedures concerns their overall impact on content area instruction. While
there have been many studies reporting the use of strategy
training for students with learning disabilities, the applicability
of such procedures to nonhandicapped students reporting
similar difficulties in secondary level learning has not routinely
appeared in the literature. Clearly, there seems to be a logical
extension possible between the self-management procedures
developed for the academic skills problems of handicapped
learners and those of nonhandicapped learners. However, few
studies, with the exception of the recently reported Esposito et
al. (1993) study, have shown how procedures such as strategy
instruction can be applied to an entire classroom of regular
education students.

In conclusion, self-management for academic skills problems still needs to be applied more broadly within the context
of regular education programs. Despite its proliferation in the
literature, it is unclear how frequently and routinely teachers
use these techniques in their instructional processes. Additional research that examines these issues is certainly needed.

NONACADEMIC SKILLS PROBLEMS

Equal attention has been given in the literature to the use of
self-management procedures to improve nonacademic school-
based behavior. Many of these procedures focus on decreasing
disruptive, or increasing appropriate, classroom behaviors. In

almost all studies, multiple component self-management packages that integrate self-monitoring, self-evaluation, and self-reinforcement are employed.

Rhode et al. (1983) described a procedure designed to increase the appropriate classroom behavior of six students with behavior disorders. In the initial phase of their study, a standard token economy system was instituted during the time students attended a resource room. At 15-minute intervals, the teacher rated each student on a 0- to 5-point scale for their behavior and academic responding during the preceding 15 minutes. Points were exchangeable at the end of the period for small toys, snacks, or special privileges. After the behavior of students improved to levels acceptable to the teacher, a self-management procedure was also implemented. Students were instructed to self-evaluate, along with their teacher, their behavioral and academic responding at the end of each 15-minute interval. Students were then given the opportunity to try and match their ratings with those of their teacher. When ratings matched exactly, students were awarded a bonus point in addition to the points they had self-assessed. If the student matched within one point, the student kept the number of points they had self-assessed. If there was more than a 1-point disagreement, the student received no points.

Over the next several phases, the matching procedure was gradually eliminated by randomly choosing only a subset of students who were required to try and match their ratings to those of the teacher. Those not involved in the matching process were allowed to keep the points they had awarded themselves that day. When the students reached the point at which no students were matching teacher ratings, complete self-management had been achieved. In this phase, surprise match periods were implemented to maintain student accuracy. Additionally, as the matching procedure was faded, the amount of time between self-assessments was lengthened to 30 minutes.

Results of the study showed consistent and strong effects across all phases. As soon as the teacher-based token-point system was instituted, all students improved their levels of appropriate behavior to 80% or better. These levels were maintained throughout all phases in which the matching procedure was in place. When the matching procedure was eliminated, appropriate behavior of the students remained at these high levels.

A particularly important aspect of the Rhode et al. (1983) study was the absence of specification for behaviors targeted for change. Instead, students were simply told the general classroom rules and were judged by the teacher as to the degree to which they followed these rules. In a sense, the students needed to learn the exact expectations of their teachers and to act accordingly. For instance, they needed to learn how to accurately determine what separated a "2" from a "3" rating by the teacher. Once this was accomplished, students could more easily adjust their own behaviors to meet the expectations of their teacher.

Smith et al. (1988) implemented a modified version of the Rhode et al. (1983) procedure in a classroom of four adolescents (13–15 years old) identified as learning disabled. These students were all found to be engaged in high levels of off-task and disruptive behaviors such as talking without permission, leaving their seat without permission, throwing objects, and interrupting the teacher during class discussions. In this study, the self-management matching procedure was implemented over a 30-minute period following baseline, without first implementing a token-point system. Initially, self-evaluation and point matching occurred every 10 minutes. This was faded to every 15 minutes and then once in 30 minutes in subsequent phases.

Results for all students were similar to the Rhode et al. (1983) study. Disruptive behavior was reduced from 60–80% of the intervals during baseline to around 20% following the beginning of the self-management program. There was a substantially greater variability in performance, however, compared with the extremely high levels of appropriate behavior noted in the Rhode et al. (1983) study.

In still another replication and extension of the Rhode et al. (1983) study, Smith, Young, Nelson, and West (1992) implemented the matching procedure with eight high school-age students identified as behavior disordered or learning disabled. In this study, their focus was on increasing on-task behavior while examining collateral changes in academic performance. Their findings were identical to previous studies, which showed that the self-management procedures resulted in substantial decreases in off-task behavior as soon as the procedures were implemented. In addition, gains in academic performance appeared to be related to the institution of the self-management program as well.

Another example of how self-management can be applied to nonacademic problems is evident in a study reported by Minner (1990). In this study, a self-monitoring procedure was used to improve the time it normally took three students with behavior disorders to walk between their resource room and regular education classrooms. The procedure involved having students press a switch that activated a stopwatch as they left one classroom and hit another switch that stopped the stopwatch upon their arrival in the second classroom. If they made the trip in the specified time, they recorded a "+" on a recording chart. Teachers also kept the time to check on the accuracy of student recording. However, students were not told on which days the teacher would be checking.

Results showed that all three students increased the percentage of the occasions they made the transitions within the criterion time from under 20% of transitions in baseline to over 80% after the intervention. Although Minner noted that the use of an electronic device might limit the adoption of such a procedure for future use, it is felt that one could obtain similar effects by having students use hand-held stopwatches. As long as teacher checking was employed, such a procedure may be a simple way to decrease time often lost in classroom transitions.

Kehle, Clark, Jenson, and Wampold (1986) reported the use of a technique known as "self-modeling" for reducing disruptive classroom behavior among students with behavior disorders. Based on the work of Dowrick and Dove (1980), this procedure involved showing students videotapes of themselves engaged in appropriate classroom behavior. These videotapes were actual footage of students, which had been edited to only include segments showing appropriate behaviors. The intervention technique simply involved requiring students to watch these videotapes for short periods of time.

In this study, three children, 10 to 13 years, were required to watch 11-minute videotapes of appropriate-only classroom behavior. Immediately after their viewing the tapes, students were observed in their classrooms for the occurrence of disruptive behaviors. Results showed that, following baseline, all three students displayed dramatic reductions in their levels of disruptive behavior. Unfortunately, a failure of disruptive behavior to return toward baseline levels upon removal of the intervention, raised some questions about the relationships between this intervention and the observed change in student behavior.

In an attempt to address some of the questions raised by Kehle et al. (1986), as well as to provide a partial replication of the effects of that study, McCurdy and Shapiro (1988) used the same technique with five students attending a self-contained school for students with serious emotional disturbance. In their study, McCurdy and Shapiro (1988) compared the effects of observing a peer or oneself modeling appropriate-only behavior, as well as attempted to control for the reactive effect of videotaping and instructions. Results of their study did not show consistent effects across students. When reductions in disruptive behavior were noted, they appeared primarily when students observed themselves rather than a peer. However, the impact of the intervention on disruptive behavior was not dramatic.

Shear and Shapiro (in press), in a further attempt to examine the impact of teaching students to self-monitor through observing appropriate-only behaviors on videotape, taught four students with behavior disorders to observe themselves using a systematic recording device. Results of this study again showed mixed effects, with only some students showing reductions in disruptive behavior.

Clark, Kehle, Jenson, and Beck (1992) have provided an excellent review of the parameters that may impact the effectiveness of self-modeling interventions. In particular, they noted that differences may be related to subject populations, target behaviors, and design considerations. At present, self-modeling appears to have a potential for altering important behavior problems in children and adolescents. However, additional research concerning its outcomes are certainly needed.

Another entire set of self-management procedures applied to nonacademic skills problems can be seen in the multitude of interventions designed for improving problem-solving skills. In particular, significant research has been conducted on teaching social skills. A large number of substantial literature reviews exist in this area and are listed in Table 2.4. A review of even a small number of these studies would be beyond the scope of this chapter. However, a general overview of the procedures used in almost all studies will be provided.

Illustrating the types of studies that have been published on the use of problem-solving training, Shapiro (1989) reported the results of a self-management program designed to teach adolescents with learning disabilities job as well as personal-related social skills aimed at improving general problem solving. These students were all seniors enrolled at vocational–technical schools.

The self-management training program developed by Shapiro and McQuillan (1986) was employed. This program consisted of 30 units that covered general self-management and problem-solving skills, as well as self-management techniques applied to job-related skills. The initial portion of the program trained students to understand their behavior in terms of antecedent–behavior–consequence relationships and how to self-identify reinforcers and use them contingently. Once these skills were learned, students were taught problem identification, goal-setting, self-monitoring, self-evaluation, and self-reinforcement. As part of the training, students were required to develop and implement personal self-management plans. Applications to problems occurring at home, at school, and on the job were incorporated into all units. Each session employed modeling, role playing, feedback, and homework assignments to teach the skills. Acquisition of the skills were assessed at 5 points during the 30-unit program through the use of brief mastery tests.

Pre- and post-test data on a problem-solving measure

TABLE 2.4. Review Articles on Social Skills Training Programs (1987–1992)

Author and date	Focus of review
Ager & Cole (1991)	Examined the use of cognitive–behavioral interventions to influence social skills and social problem solving in school-age students with behavior disorders.
Erin, Dignan, & Brown (1991)	Examined studies attempting to improve three types of social skills among children with visual impairment: assertiveness training, interactional skills, and physical communication skills.
Fine, Gilbert, Schmidt, & Haley (1989)	Reviewed studies examining use of social skills training and traditional group therapy in treating depressed adolescents.
Gaylord-Ross & Haring (1987)	Reviewed literature on improving social interaction among adolescents with severe handicaps.
Hansen, Watson-Perczel, & Christopher (1989)	Reviewed studies in terms of specific clinical issues related to social skills training with adolescents.
Hughes & Sullivan (1988)	Reviewed social skills training studies with children that used the training with social-learning or social cognitive approaches.
Inderbitzen-Pizaruk & Foster (1990)	Reviewed studies examining peer interaction and acceptance, and friendship among adolescents.
McConnell (1987)	Reviewed interventions that facilitate social interaction with regard to the concept of entrapment—a process by which the social behavior of the child comes under the control of naturally occurring reinforcers.
McEvoy & Odom (1987)	Reviewed studies on interventions for preschool children who exhibit social withdrawal or autism.
McIntosh, Vaughn, & Zaragoza (1991)	Reviewed social skills training and social interventions for children with learning disabilities.

(*continued*)

TABLE 2.4. (*Continued*)

Author and date	Focus of review
Schneider (1992)	Conducted meta-analysis of social skills training with children.
Shores (1987)	Reviewed studies on social interaction among children with behavior disorders and mental retardation. Emphasis placed on a specific program of research conducted at Vanderbilt University.
Singh, Deitz, Epstein, & Singh (1991)	Reviewed studies that attempted to improve the social behavior of children and adolescents with serious emotional disturbance.
Stern & Fodor (1989)	Reviewed studies on social skills training and interpersonal problem solving with aggressive children.
Tisdelle & St. Lawrence (1986)	Broad-based literature review on the theoretical and research-based evidence underlying interpersonal problem-solving skills.
Zaragoza, Vaughn, & McIntosh (1991)	Examined impact of social skills training on students with behavior disorders.

developed for the study were used to evaluate the impact of the training program. Results showed clear and dramatic improvements on the problem-solving measure for those students who received the self-management training compared to a nontreatment control group of adolescents with learning disabilities who did not receive the self-management program. These effects were replicated across all 3 years that the program was instituted.

Almost all programs that have been developed to teach interpersonal or job-related social skills use the same skeleton for instruction. Each begins with discussions of situations in which problem-solving skills are necessary. Students are usually encouraged to contribute examples from their own experience. Next, modeling of the appropriate way to respond in these situations is provided by the trainer (and usually a cotrainer). Modeling continues with students being asked to demonstrate and practice the targeted skills within the context of the training sessions. Substantial feedback is provided to the students by the trainers as well as their peers during this rehearsal stage. Finally, homework assignments are given to students to try and use the skills learned during sessions to events that occur in their daily lives. This approach to training can be seen in many commercially available packages such as "Skillstreaming" (Goldstein et al., 1980), "Think-Aloud" (Camp & Bash, 1985a, 1985b, 1985c), "ASSET" (Hazel, Schumaker, Sherman, & Sheldon-Wildgen, 1981), "I Can Problem Solve" (Shure, 1992a, 1992b, 1992c), as well as other developed programs.

Conclusions and Summary

From the very brief literature review presented here, it is clear that self-management procedures have broad applications for many types of nonacademic school-based problems. Improvements in the frequency of nondisruptive behavior and smooth transitions between classes, as well as the development of all types of social and problem-solving skills have been described. In each case, students were expected to assume responsibility for using the learned behaviors in settings other than those where they received training.

It should be equally clear that self-management for nonacademic skills problems can be broadly applied across various types of children and adolescents. Self-management procedures have been applicable in working with children in identified categories of special education classes, as well as with children within regular education settings, at both the young elementary and high school levels. Likewise, the procedures have been employed for difficulties experienced both within the school as well as those related to job- and community-related problems.

GENERALIZATION OF
SELF-MANAGEMENT SKILLS

One of the most often touted advantages of self-management procedures is the potential for these procedures to facilitate generalization. In particular, it is reasoned that, if the individual gains control over his or her own contingencies, he or she will be likely to use such procedures across settings, time, and activities. As such, it is anticipated that behavior change in various areas of life will become evident once self-management procedures are learned. For example, if students who self-monitor their work productivity in math experience improvements in their academic performance in that field, it is likely they will use the procedures they have learned without prompting in spelling, reading, or social studies. Thus, self-management becomes a key ingredient to establishing long-term behavior change.

Despite the logical appeal of this argument, there has been a limited empirical examination of this phenomenon. For example, Hughes, Ruhl, and Misra (1989), in a review of published literature from January 1970 through March 1988 on students identified as behaviorally disordered (or other variations of this label) who were educated in public school settings, identified a total of six studies that specifically assessed for stimulus generalization, response generalization, or generalization over time (i.e., maintenance). Those studies assessing stimulus generalization tended to examine primarily the presence of generalization across settings or persons. In those studies assessing for such changes, generalization was found. Only two studies assessed response generalization, and in one of these studies such changes were observed. All six studies assessed for maintenance, and in every case maintenance was found with upwards of 330 days of maintained response.

Fantuzzo and Polite (1990) reviewed studies from 1967 through 1988 without regard to the specific classification of disability. Their search resulted in finding 42 studies of school-based, self-management interventions targeting regular or special education classrooms. In their review, generalization was reported in a total of 18, or 43%, of these studies. These studies primarily assessed across-time and/or across-behavior generalization. In a few cases, more than one type of generalization was evaluated. Only one study assessed generalization across all possible dimensions of generalization, which showed effects across all classes of generalization.

Although there have been a smaller number of studies than expected that have actually aimed at assessing the generalized effects of self-management, the outcomes have been consistently positive. Self-management does appear to result in maintenance of behavior over time and does appear to impact change across other behaviors and tasks. However, it is of significance that in almost all the studies where generalized self-management occurred, it occurred only when the self-management procedures were specifically trained or prompted to be used in the alternative setting or with the alternative behavior. This should not be surprising, given the known variables that most likely foster generalizing behavior change (i.e., Stokes & Baer, 1977; Stokes & Osnes, 1986). It is encouraging, however, to find that self-management can produce quick and lasting change once learned.

Future studies are clearly needed that continue to provide a better and more comprehensive understanding of the dimensions under which self-management will result in generalization. However, it is also clear that achieving generalization by using self-management skills is still a process in its infancy. Further, additional efforts need to be made at demonstrating the generalizability of these skills.

GENERAL CONCLUSIONS FROM RESEARCH

What has the research taught us about self-management? As should be evident from this brief and certainly abridged review, self-management encompasses a very powerful set of techniques, which can be applied broadly across ages, populations, and types of problems. It can have widespread application to all types of academic skills, ranging from preschool match-to-sample tasks to content area instruction in biology. It can provide a means for improving nonacademic behaviors such as transition time between classes and out-of-seat behavior, as well as complex behavioral responses such as problem-solving skills and job-related social skills.

With little question, the research support for using self-management in the schools is clear and unequivocal. Interestingly, we know little about how much self-management is actually being used, and about how acceptable such a procedure really is to teachers, students, and parents. As noted by Fantuzzo and Polite (1990) in their review of 42 studies, only two ever assessed social validity. Likewise, significant questions remain about the use of self-management as a tool to achieve generalization. What are the limits of self-management generalization? How many prompts are needed across settings or tasks before students begin using these procedures on their own? Are students with particular behavioral or personality characteristics better candidates for self-management interventions than others? These are important and, as yet, unanswered questions.

Clearly, there is a strong interest among researchers in the area of self-management. Indeed, the logical and philosophical appeal of providing intervention strategies that result in personal behavior change and increased student self-responsibility are the desire of any educator. Continued research into the mechanisms and impact of self-management is still needed.

3

Intervention: Contingency-Based Approaches

As discussed in Chapter 1, self-management interventions can be roughly divided into those procedures that are based on contingency management and those that are based on cognitive control. In this chapter, descriptions of several contingency-based self-management interventions will be provided. By no means should the types of procedures described nor their particular applications to specific problems be viewed as exhaustive. Instead, these should be viewed as illustrative of the many ways that self-management can be applied in classroom settings. Further, practitioners should regard the material as having easy applicability to different types of academic or behavior problems, different populations of students, and different age levels.

As one examines these procedures, it is also important to recognize that it is often impossible to separate self-monitoring procedures from those that also incorporate self-evaluation and self-reinforcement components. While some interventions presented here contain only self-monitoring as a primary intervention, many others incorporate several components of self-management. For the sake of clarity, those procedures that emphasize self-monitoring alone will be discussed independent of procedures that incorporate self-monitoring plus additional components of self-management.

SELF-MONITORING: BASIC METHODS

The methodology of self-monitoring is really rather simple. Once a behavior is specified, the student is taught to record the occurrence of that behavior without prompting from others. Recording devices can vary greatly and can include simple pencil-and-paper methods of recording a tick mark for each occurrence of a behavior. Figure 3.1 offers illustrations of some different types of recording devices. In addition to pencil-and-paper methods, one can use mechanical recording devices such as response counters when self-monitoring. Students have also used specially made devices for self-monitoring when they do not have the cognitive capacity to count. For example, Shapiro et al. (1984), in working with young autistic students who lacked numeration skills, developed a device that contained five holes into which plastic tokens could be placed. Students were taught to self-monitor the completion of worksheets by placing a token from a container into one of the holes upon finishing their work. When all of the holes were filled, the students were said to meet the criteria set by the teacher for work finished that day.

In its simplest form, self-monitoring requires a student to self-observe that a specified behavior has occurred and to record its occurrence in some way. The use of additional backup reinforcers or procedures to evaluate the accuracy of the recording may be unnecessary. Just having students engage in self-monitoring may provide a powerful and useful mechanism for behavior change.

SELF-MONITORING: APPLICATIONS TO ATTENTIONAL BEHAVIOR PROBLEMS

The procedure for applying self-monitoring to attentional, or on-task, behavior involves providing a cueing mechanism for students and having them determine if they have or have not

YES	NO

TALKING	NO TALKING

STUDY RECORD
Name: _____ Date: _____
Record a "+" if you were studying.
Record a "–" if you were not studying.

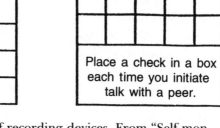

Place a check in a box
each time you initiate
talk with a peer.

FIGURE 3.1. Examples of self-recording devices. From "Self-monitoring Procedures" in *Behavioral Assessment in Schools: Conceptual Foundations and Practical Applications* (p. 213) by E. S. Shapiro & T. R. Kratochwill (Eds.), 1988, New York, Guilford Press. Copyright 1988 by Guilford Press. Reprinted by permission.

been engaging in on-task behavior at the moment the cue was given. Most often, the cueing mechanism is an audiotaped signal. Students are trained to ask themselves the question, "Was I paying attention?" at the sound of the tone. Each student then records in some way whether or not he or she was paying attention.

Hallahan et al. (1981) provided a good prototype for this type of self-monitoring procedure, which involved the following sequence:

1. Students were given response counters to be worn on their wrists that could record the occurrence of each self-monitored behavior.
2. A tape recording was played that provided audible beeps randomly from 10–90 seconds apart. The beeps occurred on average every 45 seconds.
3. At the occurrence of each tone, students were instructed to ask themselves, "Was I paying attention when I heard the beep?" They were told to press their response counter if the answer to that self-asked question was a "Yes," and not to press the counter if their answer was a "No."
4. Students were trained over a 3-day period. To ensure that students accurately discriminated on- from off-task behavior, role playing and the modeling of on- and off-task behavior by the teacher was used. Students then also modeled and role played the self-monitoring activity.
5. After it was found that the self-monitoring procedure could substantially increase on-task behavior, the use of the wrist counters was faded by telling students to continue keeping track of their on- and off-task behavior when they heard the tone, but not to record their behavior by pushing a response counter.
6. The use of the tape recorded cueing was also faded once students showed that they did not need to use a response counter to maintain high levels of on-task behavior.

An important aspect of this procedure was that no additional backup rewards were applied. Students were only provided with the reinforcers naturally present in classrooms for completing their assigned work (i.e., better grades, positive attention from the teacher and parents, more positive classroom attitudes). Use of these procedures with multiple students simultaneously is obviously possible. In fact, as a classwide intervention procedure, this technique can be quite effective.

Considerations in Using Self-Monitoring for Attentional Behavior Problems

In using this type of procedure for improving the on-task behavior of students, several elements must be taken into consideration. First, the use of a tape recorded cueing device can be potentially distracting to students. When implementing these procedures, some students will spend much of their time waiting for the tape recorded signal rather than working on their assigned activities. These students are often highly distractible and unable to both work and attend to an auditory signal simultaneously.

Second, some children become highly engaged in their assigned activity and forget to self-monitor. Thus, the accuracy of their self-monitoring remains poor, yet they show substantial improvements in on-task behavior because of the implementation of the procedure. It is important that teachers do not insist on 100% accurate self-monitoring if the procedure results in sustained attention to task.

Third, when the procedure is used with only a subset of students in a classroom, it is often necessary to provide them with an earphone connection to a tape recorder to prevent the audio cue from distracting others in the classroom who do not need such individualized intervention. Indeed, this technique can be very effective in helping a student who is receiving instructions in a setting with other students not experiencing on-task problems simply by using a personal audio cueing device.

Fourth, students sometimes do not effectively discriminate on- from off-task behavior. That is, they may be off-task at the moment the cue sounds, but then begin working immediately after hearing the tone. Thus, they record themselves as on-task for that cued interval. It is important that students be taught to discriminate working from not working during the training. Learning this difference should be reinforced throughout the intervention, until the student attains a very high level of on-task behavior.

Fifth, students need to have a clear idea of the required behavior. For many students, on- and off-task behaviors are simple to understand, and easily defined by using the terms "working" and "not working." It is helpful, however, if the student is reminded periodically of what is defined as "working." This is especially important when the tasks change from independent seatwork to more discussion-oriented, teacher-directed activities.

Another issue that sometimes emerges is the failure of students to remain interested in the intervention after a period of time. One solution that may be helpful is to alter the audio cueing from beeps to other sounds. One can use bells, whistles, sirens, funny noises, and other such cues to keep the student interested in the technique. Musical interludes of 5–10 seconds of popular recordings have also been used as an alternative to beeps. This is often a very motivating procedure for students who are highly distractible and easily bored with other intervention techniques.

A very critical aspect of the intervention is the use of cues played at random intervals. The purpose of the randomization of intervals is to prevent the student from accurately predicting when the next cue will occur. By randomly inserting cues from as close as 10 seconds apart to as far as 90 seconds apart, sustained levels of on-task performance are likely to be achieved. It is important that the intervals are not played at consistent time periods (such as every 30 seconds). This will likely result in students learning to work on a fixed-interval schedule. Hence, they will often stop working for about 25 seconds between intervals.

Modifications of Self-Monitoring Procedures for Attentional Behavior Problems

One modification of the self-monitoring procedure described above is to not include any cueing procedure at all. As noted in several of the studies discussed in Chapter 2, some researchers have found successful outcomes by simply providing students with a paper-and-pencil recording device and telling them to "record themselves as working or not working whenever they felt like it." As unlikely as it seems that such a procedure would result in behavior change, enough successful studies have been reported in the literature to suggest that such a procedure can work for some students (e.g., McLaughlin, 1984; Piersel, 1985).

Another modification of the procedure described by Hallahan et al. (1981) has been to use visual prompting devices, as opposed to audiotones, to remind students of the requirements for on-task behavior. Figure 3.2 shows an example of a cueing device used by Prater et al. (1991). Her procedure involved using a paper-and-pencil self-recording device along with audio cueing, which occurred between 1 and 2.5 minutes across different students. Fading procedures incorporated the removal of the audiotones but maintenance of the visual prompting procedures. Use of such visual prompters can promote the long-term maintenance of this type of behavior.

Other modifications of the procedures have involved altering the amount of delay between audio cues. There are no specific criteria for whether one should use cues on an average of every 15, 30, 45, or 60 seconds. In general, most studies

REMEMBER:

(1) Eyes on teacher or on work

(2) Sitting in seat
Facing forward
Feet on floor or legs crossed

(3) Using correct materials

(4) Working silently

FIGURE 3.2. Example of a visual cueing device. From "Self-Monitoring of On-Task Behavior by Adolescents with Learning Disabilities" by M. A. Prater, R. Joy, B. Chilman, J. Temple, S. R. Miller, 1991, *Learning Disability Quarterly, 14,* p. 169. Copyright 1991 by Council for Learning Disabilities. Reprinted by permission.

reported using this procedure have employed average interval lengths of between 45 and 120 seconds. Our suggestion is to begin with a shorter interval if the student is highly distractible in the beginning and gradually lengthen the interval as behavior improves.

One additional modification that has been made frequently is the addition of a back-up reinforcer when self-monitoring alone does not result in behavior change. This is done by establishing a criteria for performance before students begin the intervention. If the criteria is met, students earn their chosen rewards. A possible problem that can emerge when using this procedure is that if, during the work period, a student recognizes that his or her behavior cannot possibly meet the preestablished criteria, he or she may stop working all together. A technique that addresses this problem is known as the "mystery motivator" (Moore, Waguespack, Wickstrom, Witt, & Gaydos, in press; Rhode, Jenson, & Reavis, 1992). The "mystery-motivator" procedure involves having the teacher write the preset criteria for accomplishing a task on a piece of paper, and then place it in an envelope to be attached to a blackboard. When the intervention period is finished, the envelope is opened and the results announced. Students then compare their performance against the mystery criteria and gain access to the rewards according to how close the two match. In this way, the student cannot predict the criteria for performance before they complete their work. The teacher can likewise manipulate the student level of performance by varying the criteria so that they are always different, sometimes establishing a very low level so that all students will be likely to meet it, and sometimes a very high level that only a few can meet. This procedure has been found to be a very exciting and highly motivating technique, especially for younger children.

SELF-MONITORING: APPLICATIONS TO ACADEMIC BEHAVIOR

Self-monitoring procedures have often been applied to the management of academic responses. Academic subjects such as reading comprehension, spelling, creative writing, or math computation have been targeted, as well as the level of academic productivity such as work or homework completion. The procedures used derive from the basic self-monitoring procedure used to improve on-task behavior that was described in the previous section.

Lalli and Shapiro (1990) describe the use of self-monitoring in the acquisition of "sight" word vocabulary. The procedure involved the following steps:

1. Lists of 15 unknown words were developed from pre-baseline assessments of words taken from the student's basal reading material.
2. Audiotapes were prepared with words read at 5-second intervals.
3. The student was instructed to read words aloud from prepared lists as the tape recorder was played. Immediately after reading the word aloud, the student would hear the word read on the tape recorder and was taught to mark a "+" or "−" according to whether he or she had read the word correctly or incorrectly. The student was taught that a word was considered incorrect if he or she could not finish reading it before he or she began hearing the word on the tape recording.
4. The total words read correct and incorrect were tallied by the student at the end of the session.

The procedure used by Lalli and Shapiro (1990) offers an excellent and simple method for students to practice learning words. The same procedure could easily be applied to math facts or other such fact-based learning. Rewards based on meeting preset criteria could also be added to the procedure.

Another procedure involves the self-management of spelling performance. Again, using audiotape recorders, the procedure can be set up so that all drill and practice, as well as examination, activities can be employed by the students themselves.

The procedure requires the development of two sets of

audiotapes: one to be used for practice and the other for testing. Here are the details of the procedure:

1. Generate two word lists on audiotape:
   a. List 1 (*practice*): SAY the word, WAIT 7–10 seconds, SPELL the word. (Teacher can use a sentence to illustrate use of the word if desired during the 7–10-second wait period.)
   b. List 2 (*test*): SAY the word, WAIT 7–10 seconds, SAY the next word. (Teacher can use a sentence to illustrate use of the word if desired during the 7–10-second wait period.)

   Lists can be taken from weekly spelling list assignments, or can be teacher generated.

2. Student practice sessions:
   a. Provide student with prepared sheet for spelling practice (see Figure 3.3).
   b. Student turns on practice tape. When they hear each word, they are instructed to do the following in the order given:
      • Turn off the tape recorder
      • Write the word on the first column
      • Turn on the tape recorder
      • Write the word again as you hear it spelled correctly on the tape
      • Check your spelling against the correct spelling
      • If correct, go to the next word
      • If incorrect, turn off the tape recorder and write the correct spelling three times across the next three columns
   c. When finished, the student records the number correct on the first try as well as the percentage of words correct.
   d. Results are graphed.
   e. When a student scores 100% on practice, he or she is ready to be tested on the word list.

3. Student test sessions
   a. Student obtains prepared sheet for test session (see Figure 3.4).

Spelling Practice

Name: _____
Date: _____
Spelling Unit #: _____

Word #	Your Spelling	Correct Spelling	Right? Y/N	Correct #1	Correct #2	Correct #3
1						
2						
3						
4						
5						
6						
7						
8						
9						
10						
11						
12						
13						
14						
15						

FIGURE 3.3. Self-monitoring sheet for spelling practice.

Spelling Test

Name : _____
Date: _____
Spelling Unit #: _____

Word #	Your Spelling	Right? Y/N	Correct #1	Correct #2	Correct #3
1					
2					
3					
4					
5					
6					
7					
8					
9					
10					
11					
12					
13					
14					
15					

FIGURE 3.4. Self-monitoring sheet for spelling test.

    b. Student turns on tape. When he or she hears a word he or she is instructed to:
- Write the word (with or without turning off the tape, as the teacher chooses)
- Go to the next word
- When finished, check your spelling against the spelling list (provided by the teacher or from a spelling book)
- Write any incorrect words three times in the space provided on the test sheet

    c. Results are scored and graphed.

    d. If score is greater than teacher-established criteria (85% is suggested), the student goes to the next spelling practice list.

    e. If score is less than established criteria, student is instructed to continue practice sessions again until 100% is obtained. Test is then retaken.

The procedure described above provides an opportunity for students to completely self-manage their practicing and testing for spelling performance. Further, the procedure can allow a student to progress through material at an individualized pace. In addition, the drill and practice activities can be done as supplements to the existing spelling drills provided in the spelling curriculum materials, or it can supplant some of the materials.

Certain questions are often raised by teachers who use this procedure. For example, they wonder whether students will cheat during the practice sessions, by simply waiting for the correct spelling rather than writing down their spelling attempt. While it is certainly true that students can do this since the procedures are implemented under conditions of self-management, it is also likely that they will be unsuccessful on the exam that tests what they have learned. Thus, they will have to recycle several times back to the practice sessions in order to meet the criteria necessary to move on. It should not take long before students realize the value, importance, and efficiency in completing the practice activities as prescribed.

Teachers also wonder if students will progress through

materials too quickly. They sometimes become concerned that the emphasis of these drill and test activities is on memorization rather than on understanding the phonetic characteristics of the words which are the focus of drills appearing in the spelling curriculum. Again, it is not suggested that this self-management procedure should replace all spelling activities normally provided in the instructional sequence. Indeed, for many students a procedure such as this is unnecessary. However, for the student who fails to succeed in spelling despite routinely following the best instructional practices, the self-management spelling procedure described here can provide a valuable and important adjunct to regular instruction.

Teachers also wonder about the amount of time and effort needed to generate audiotapes of spelling lists. While we have not found the procedures to be highly time consuming, we have, at times, used other students to develop the audiotapes for peers. In some cases, we have even suggested to the student who will use the technique to develop the audiotapes him- or herself. This, of course, requires that the student has sufficient reading skills to be able to read a spelling list accurately.

The procedure described for spelling could be easily adapted for many other drill activities. It could be applied to simple activities like the acquisition of math facts or multiplication tables, or more complex tasks like learning the vocabulary of a biology textbook. Again, the procedures are the same, only the content of material is altered.

Lam et al. (in press) described a procedure for self-monitoring academic accuracy in math computation. While working on a worksheet containing problems that were selected for the individual student based on his or her preassessed level of mastery, an audio tone was played at approximately 1-minute intervals. Upon hearing the tone, the student was taught to mark the problem on which he or she was working, move the cover sheet downward to check his or her answers since the previous tone had been heard, and then to write the number of problems correct in the right hand margin where indicated. This procedure combined the cued self-monitoring technique described previously with a self-monitoring for academic accuracy.

Although others have used simpler techniques for self-monitoring academic accuracy with success, such as having students self-record their correct responses after completing an entire worksheet of problems, the technique described by Lam et al. (in press) is unique in that students self-monitored throughout the instructional period. This is important especially for students who may be likely to make numerous errors before the implementation of the self-monitoring period. If a student waits until all problems have been attempted before self-monitoring, he or she may lose a valuable opportunity to receive feedback closer in time to the actual occurrence of the error.

In a type of self-management procedure also designed to offer a student immediate feedback for their performance, Skinner et al. (1989) described a procedure called "Cover, Copy, and Compare," which helps students acquire mathematical computational skills. The procedure requires students to engage in a specific academic response, immediately compare their response to the correct answer, and to record if their answer was correct. The procedure incorporates self-assessment, self-recording, and self-evaluation.

Specifically, the procedure used for improving addition performance involves the following steps:

1. Students are given a sheet of math problems with the problems and their answers listed in a column on the left hand side of the paper (see Figure 3.5).
2. Students are instructed to look at the first problem and its answer.
3. Students then cover the answer with a piece of construction paper.
4. Students then write the problem and answer on the right hand side of the original math problems.
5. Students uncover the problem and evaluate if their answer was correct.
6. If correct, students place a "+" mark next to the problem.
7. If incorrect, students repeat the procedure until they respond correctly.

Look	Cover	Copy	Compare: + if Correct
5 +3 ─── 8			
4 +2 ─── 6			
6 +1 ─── 7			
5 +2 ─── 7			
3 +4 ─── 7			
8 +1 ─── 9			
3 +3 ─── 6			
2 +2 ─── 4			

FIGURE 3.5. Cover, Copy, Compare worksheet.

The procedure has many advantages. It provides students with immediate, corrective feedback as soon as they respond. Further, the technique can easily be applied to almost any subject area. As a self-management strategy, students can learn to apply the intervention with only minimal training and can be completely self-directed. In particular, the procedure may have substantial advantages for students who need to learn specific techniques for improving study skills.

SELF-MANAGEMENT: APPLICATIONS WITH NONACADEMIC SKILLS PROBLEMS

The procedures and techniques already discussed for academic and attentional problems, can be applied to nonacademic skills problems with equal success. As long as the behavior is specified and the student trained in using the technique, self-monitoring can easily be used for a wide range of different behavior problems. In general, when self-management is used for nonacademic skills or behavior problems that don't involve attention to task, the procedures incorporate multiple components of self-management. Typically, methods include self-monitoring and self-evaluation. Often, self-reinforcement procedures are also added to the self-management package. While many applications of self-management to disruptive or nonacademic skills problems can be found, the techniques described in detail by Rhode et al. (1983) provide perhaps the best approach to developing effective self-management techniques for these types of behavior problems. Indeed, the procedures described by Rhode et al. (1983) have been replicated with success several times in studies reported by Smith et al. (1992), Smith et al. (1988), and Young, Smith, West, and Morgan (1987). In addition, the procedures have been implemented with young children as well as adolescents.

Using a Self-Evaluation Procedure

The Rhode et al. procedure involves two phases. In the initial phase, students are taught the processes of self-monitoring and self-evaluation. Typically, the processes are implemented first with a small number of children under the direct supervision of a teacher well-skilled in using behavioral intervention techniques. This might commonly be a special education teacher. The self-management strategy is taught within the confines of a restricted setting and for a restricted time period, in order for students to learn the basic concepts of self-management. Once learned under these conditions, however, the procedure is very easy to transport to other settings, time periods, and academic subjects. As such, the procedure becomes ideal for use in mainstream classroom settings. Here are the steps in implementing this self-management intervention technique:

Phase 1: Resource room or other similar setting

1. *Step 1: Token reinforcement/systematic feedback.* The primary objective of this step of the procedure is to provide a mechanism for teachers to provide frequent and meaningful feedback to students using numerical information. The step involves the following procedure:
   a. Classroom rules posted by teacher.
   b. At 15-minute intervals signaled by a timer, the teacher awards each student points based on the teacher's judged rating of his or her academic and behavioral performance.
   c. Teacher ratings at 15-minute intervals are given on a 0–5-point scale for behavior and academic performance, with a total of up to 10 possible points. Teachers are given the following guidelines for making point awards:
      • 5—Excellent (all classroom rules followed for entire 15-minute interval; all work done with 100% accuracy).
      • 4—Very good (minor rule infractions occasionally; worked almost entire interval with work being at least 90% correct).
      • 3—Average (broke one or more rules to extent that behavior was not acceptable; followed rules

> 80% of the time; work completed with 70–80% accuracy).
> - 2—Below average (broke one or more rules to extent that behavior was not acceptable, but followed rules part of the time; work completed with 60–80% accuracy).
> - 1—Poor (broke one or more rules most of the period; high degree of inappropriate behavior; work was less than 60% accurate).
> - 0—Totally unacceptable (broke one or more rules for entire interval; did not work at all; most work was incorrect).

Using these guidelines, teachers rate each student on a 0–5 scale for academic performance and a 0–5 scale for their behavior. Although the guidelines are provided, it is suggested to teachers that they simply try to be consistent in their ratings over time. It is not necessary for teachers to actually assess whether students were 80–90% accurate or only violated one rule. What is important is that teachers remain consistent in their ratings over time. The teacher's ratings are told to each student individually at the end of each 15-minute interval. A brief verbal explanation for ratings are also given.

2. *Step 2: Matching student self-evaluation with teacher with 100% of the students.* Once the students' behavior during Step 1 has improved to a level that the teacher finds acceptable, and there has been sufficient time for the teacher to establish consistency in the ratings of the students, Step 2 begins. The purpose of Step 2 is to have students begin the process of conducting self-evaluations, as well as examining the degree to which their self-evaluations match those of their teachers.
   a. Students rate themselves on behavior and academic performance after each 15-minute interval.
   b. Teachers continue to rate the students also, independently of the student self-evaluations.
   c. Ratings of students and teachers are compared. Stu-

dents provide brief verbal explanations for why they gave themselves a particular rating.

d. If students match within one point of their teachers' ratings, they get to keep the number of points they awarded themselves.

e. If a student's rating is exactly the same as that of the teacher, the student is awarded a bonus point.

f. If a student's rating is off by more than one point, he or she earns no points for that interval.

g. All students in the class engaged in using the self-management procedure are permitted the opportunity to earn bonus points through matching.

This procedure provides a mechanism for students to try and learn the process of self-evaluation *based on the expected level of behavior of their teacher.*

3. *Step 3: Elimination of matching with 50% of the students.* Once the students establish high and acceptable levels of accuracy while maintaining minimal disruptiveness, the matching procedure is systematically eliminated.

a. Students continue to self-evaluate at the end of each 15-minute interval along with the teacher.

b. At the end of each 15-minute interval, all of the students' names are placed into a bowl and half of them are randomly selected. Only the students selected are permitted to match the teacher's ratings for bonus points.

c. Students not matching are permitted to keep the points they awarded themselves, regardless of the teacher ratings they received.

d. Brief verbal discussions about the reasons for self-awarded points are held with each student.

4. *Steps 4, 5, 6: Elimination of matching with 33 1/3%, 16 2/3%, 0% of the students.* Through the next series of steps, the number of students permitted to match with the teacher is divided in half for each step. In addition, the rating interval is gradually lengthened first to every 20 minutes and then to every 30 minutes. In order to

ensure that students are unlikely to cheat during this process, the teacher occasionally conducts a "surprise match" for all students during various intervals.

At this step in the procedure, the students have learned an effective method for self-management within the confines of a small classroom for a specific subject and with a specific teacher. The second phase of the procedure involves using the procedure across settings, teachers, time, and/or subject matter. The exact way that one takes the procedure and extends it varies according to the needs of the student. In the example described below, the procedure involves extending the technique to a mainstream, regular classroom setting.

Phase 2: Generalization to regular setting

1. *Step 1: Self-evaluation in a regular classroom setting (every 30 minutes).* In this step of the procedure, the same types of ratings that were previously described are implemented in a regular classroom setting. At the end of each 30-minute period, the teacher and student are rated on a 0–5 point scale for academic and behavioral performance. These ratings are recorded on an index card to be carried by the student. At a designated time, the student meets with the special education teacher to determine whether he or she has accurately rated him- or herself, and points are awarded.
2. *Step 2: Fading of self-evaluation.* Over the next phase, the entire self-evaluation procedure is faded.
   a. Intervals between self-ratings are extended to 60 minutes.
   b. Point exchange occurs at the end of the day instead of at midday.
3. *Step 3: Fading of point exchange.* During this step, the point exchange for backup rewards is gradually eliminated.
   a. Point exchange is made variable across days.
   b. Students are not informed until after the session if the point exchange is to be made on that day.

      c. Surprise matches during the week are used as needed.

4. *Step 4: Eliminate point exchange, fade self-evaluation.* During this step, the point exchange is completely eliminated and students begin the process of moving from written self-evaluation to more covert forms of self-evaluation.

      a. Students no longer mark ratings on their cards.

      b. Verbal feedback continues from the teacher and students.

      c. Verbal feedback now used every 2 days on a random schedule.

5. *Step 5: Student self-management.* The final phase includes no verbal or written feedback on student performance. Students are told to continue to keep track of their performance "to themselves."

Considerations in Using the Self-Evaluation Procedure

In using the self-evaluation procedure just described, several important factors must be considered. First, if during the fading procedures, classroom-appropriate behavior drops below teacher expectations on 3 consecutive days, then booster sessions of 10–15 minutes on following the rules are implemented. During these sessions, students return to steps in the procedure in which complete rating and matching against teacher ratings is used 100% of the time. Second, the procedure described can be modified in several ways. Here are several questions often asked in setting up programs that use this procedure, with corresponding responses:

    Do teachers have to rate students every 15 minutes? A frequent concern raised by teachers in using this procedure is the need for such frequent feedback to students about their behavior. Indeed, 15-minute ratings may be viewed as excessive and possibly unnecessary. There is no magic about using 15-minute intervals. The procedure has been used successfully when teachers and students conduct ratings on academic subjects (i.e., reading, math, social studies) at 30-minute intervals, before lunch and before leaving school only, as well as every 10 minutes. In truth, the interval between rating sessions depends on the needs of the student. For some students, every 15 minutes is too often and highly distracting. For others, it is too short. It is perfectly acceptable to experiment with the procedure until one finds an interval that works for the students with whom it is being implemented.

Can this procedure be done without having the teacher rate behavior before the student? Of course you can start the procedure by having the student and teacher simultaneously rate behavior. Sometimes this approach does not work as well since students must take some time to learn how to judge their behavior in view of the teacher's perceptions. That is, the advantage to having a phase where the teacher alone rates the student's behavior, offers the student an opportunity to learn the relationship between their actions and the teacher's judgment of these actions. Once learned, it becomes easier for students to accurately match the teacher's expectations through their own behavioral ratings. In general, it is recommended that a period of time be implemented when the teacher does the rating alone and communicates the results to the student.

Is the use of backup rewards necessary? No, it is not always necessary to use backup rewards. Teachers need to experiment with the potential effects the procedure will have without such rewards to determine if the technique is successful without them.

How long do I use the procedure in one classroom before using it in other regular education settings? If one is using the procedure for the purpose of trying to promote improvement across settings, it is important that the student clearly learn the expectations (as reflected in the ratings) of the teacher within one classroom. Once it is clear that the student can consistently rate themselves accurately, using the procedure in other regular classroom settings is usually easy. Indeed, because the student understands the procedure and has been successful with it, using it in other classrooms simply requires the student to begin to learn the behavioral expectations of other teachers, as reflected in their ratings. This usually does not take very much time.

What if the student is not in a special education setting? It is certainly possible to use this procedure entirely within the mainstream environment. What is important, however, is that the matching procedure be implemented under controlled conditions before it is used on a widespread basis across a student's academic day. For example, if the procedure were to be used within a mainstream environment alone, one might first implement self-management only during a single 45-minute math period each day. In this way, the student can learn the requirements of the intervention and become effective at accurately rating his or her own behavior before being asked to do this throughout the day. Likewise, this gives the teacher a chance to become comfortable with the techniques as well as work out any unforeseen "bugs" that may arise in trying to use the self-management program. Once the student has learned how to engage in self-management within the 45-minute math period, use of the procedure can be quickly added to other parts of the instructional day.

Can this procedure be used with parents as well as teachers? Absolutely. The technique is a generic self-management package that can be applied across any setting, subject, or set of individuals. In using the procedure with parents, it is important that the time periods for evaluation be clearly established, and that the parents only rate the child based on what they can observe. If their child disrupts a playground activity outside the observational possibilities of the parents, they should not rate him or her poorly because of the reports of others.

Do teachers need to do this procedure for more than 60 minutes per day? The answer to this question depends on the student's responsiveness to the technique. The procedure needs to be done for a long enough period of time so that the student can make several self-ratings. This may require only an hour or it may require several hours. Again, the basic concepts of self-management can be applied and adapted to the needs of the situation presented to the teacher.

Other Examples of Self-Management for Nonacademic Skills Problems

One of the problems often faced by psychologists and other consultants in working with students with behavior problems is that many times the student is unaware him- or herself of the presence of inappropriate behavior. Shapiro, Albright, and Ager (1986) describe the use of a self-monitoring procedure to reduce the inappropriate verbalizations of a 14-year-old girl who failed to acknowledge the presence of her inappropriate behavior. The procedure involved targeting high-frequency, negative actions, such as using sarcasm, calling out obscenities, or using a loud or rude tone of voice. The researchers decided to set up a procedure where the girl would monitor positive and appropriate verbalizations, which were defined as any response to directions, consequences, or conversation in which positive words, tone of voice, and appropriate facial expressions were used, and which did not include the use of sarcasm, obscenities, a loud or rude tone of voice, or obscene gestures. With the girl's behavioral patterns, it was not possible to count discrete occurrences of single behaviors, hence episodes of behavioral responding were counted instead. Episodes ended after 1 minute of noninteraction, which was defined as 1 minute of nontalking.

Following baseline data collection, a self-monitoring procedure was implemented. After explaining to the student how the teacher defined the problem behavior, the student was instructed to make a tally mark on a card each time she engaged in a verbalization involving a response to a teacher or peer request, and to mark if the verbalization was appropriate. At the same time, the teacher or an observer in the classroom, also tallied the number of appropriate verbalizations. If the girl's total number of appropriate verbalizations at the end of the day equaled 95% or better of the observer's tally, the student was rewarded by being permitted to leave school 5 minutes earlier than normal. In this example, the student was only required to match the teacher's recording. There were no set criteria for her performance.

The reason the goal was accurate self-monitoring is the

student often refused to acknowledge that she had actually engaged in inappropriate verbalizations. As such, it was decided to start the procedure by asking her to achieve accuracy in her self-monitoring and, if that failed to change her behavior, then to implement set criteria for performance.

Results of the study showed that achieving accurate recording significantly improved her rate of appropriate verbalizations. The simple procedure of asking the student to record and try to match the teacher's ratings again proved to be a powerful tool in achieving sustained behavior change.

CONCLUSIONS

It should be very clear that the use of self-management is no different than the use of any other behaviorally oriented, contingency-management procedure. Similar to the awarding of points by the teacher following occurrences of desired behaviors in a token economy, the implementation of self-management procedures follows identical principles. After a response occurs, the behavior is recorded, evaluated, and rewarded if it meets the prestated criterion. This procedure can clearly be applied whether the child's problem is the completion of his or her homework, the accurate calculation of math problems, excessive calling out during classroom discussions, or a frequent use of abusive language. The key differences from other contingency-management approaches, of course, is that the student him- or herself is responsible for the implementation of the recording, evaluating, and rewarding. This shift from control by others to self-control is a critical and essential component for effective and lasting behavior change.

The procedures used to provide contingency-based self-management are fairly simple and straightforward. Yet, they have been found to have significant impact when used as prescribed. It is important that one is not deceived by their simplicity. Although the procedures look easy to put in place, they require a shift in the thinking of the teacher or parent. They require that teachers or parents recognize the need for students to control their own behavior and take responsibility for their actions.

It is also important to recognize that the examples provided in this chapter only represent a small portion of the possible ways that self-management procedures can be used. Interested readers are encouraged to use their imagination in reasoning how a specific problem presented in a classroom might be solved by using one or a combination of the many self-management techniques described.

4

Intervention: Cognitive-Based Approaches

With the emergence and evolution of cognitive behavior therapy over the past two decades, cognitive-based interventions have been developed for a wide variety of academic and emotional/behavior problems presented by children and adolescents. Cognitive-based self-management interventions are a heterogeneous group of procedures, which overlap considerably with other cognitive and noncognitive approaches. However, they all share the central assumption that a child's behavior and emotions primarily result from how environmental events are perceived by him or her. The implication for intervention is that problem behaviors can be improved by somehow changing the way the child views events in his or her world.

More simply stated, these strategies are designed to teach children to think differently about a situation before they act. For example, an academically competent child who is off-task a great deal of the day may be thinking negative thoughts that perpetuate task avoidance (e.g., "Why do I have to do this," "This is dumb," or "I hate school"). Teaching this child to approach tasks using positive, self-instructional statements may result in improved attendance and academic performance. It is important to note, however, that the addition of cognitive concepts does not imply an abandonment of those contingency-based procedures typically associated with the behavioral approach. Rather, it merely represents a shift away from sole reliance on external environmental events to an additional consideration of what the child is thinking and feeling in a particular context. The aim is to focus more on the antecedents for appropriate behavior than on external consequences for appropriate or inappropriate actions.

The target behaviors that are measured may be similar to those contingency-based approaches confront. However, the focus of the intervention is different. With cognitive-based interventions, the child is taught to employ specific self-instructions, cognitions, or problem-solving strategies that may lead him or her to engage in self-monitoring, self-evaluation, and self-reinforcement. The approach attempts to first alter mediational processes that hopefully will lead to self-managed behavior.

Mahoney and Arnkoff (1978) have identified three major forms of cognitive-based interventions: rational approaches, coping-skills approaches, and problem-solving approaches. These categories are expanded upon in Table 4.1. One variation of a rational approach that is popular for use with children is self-instruction training (Meichenbaum, 1977). In this approach, children are taught to talk to themselves in an effort to modify their problem behavior. The second major form of cognitive-based interventions identified by Mahoney and Arnkoff (1978) is termed coping-skills approaches. Although this category overlaps considerably with rational approaches such as self-instruction training, the distinguishing feature of this class of interventions is that the student learns to cope with

TABLE 4.1. Cognitive-Based Interventions

Major categories	Examples of specific procedures
Rational approaches	Self-instruction training
Coping-skills approaches	Stress inoculation training
Problem-solving approaches	Social problem-solving training, social skills training

stress-producing situations (Wilson, 1978). An example of a coping-skills approach to be discussed in this chapter is stress inoculation training (Meichenbaum, 1977). Finally, problem-solving approaches represent the third major form of cognitive-based interventions. As in the case of the coping-skills approaches, this category includes a heterogeneous group of procedures that overlap with a variety of other approaches. Specific approaches discussed here include social problem-solving and social skills training programs, each of which has been used in a variety of settings with children and adolescents presenting various difficulties.

SELF-INSTRUCTION TRAINING

Description

The primary goal of self-instruction training is to teach the child verbal behavior that will help guide his or her nonverbal actions. For example, a child may be taught verbalizations that will help successfully direct her through an academic task. Or, a student with a history of fighting on the playground may be taught to engage in self-instructional statements when teased by peers. With this approach, the academic or behavior problems exhibited by many children are assumed to reflect deficits in the ability to mediate behavior. Problems are thought to result from impulsive, nonreflective responding. The intervention implication of this assumption is that, if children can be taught self-talk behaviors designed to initiate, direct, or redirect their behavior, academic and/or behavior problems may be eliminated.

Background

Self-instruction training was developed in the late 1960s and early 1970s by Meichenbaum. In conceptualizing self-instruction training, he drew from the writings of the Soviet psychologists Luria (1961) and Vygotsky (1962). These writers proposed a developmental model of self-control consisting of three stages by which children's voluntary motor behaviors would come under verbal control. They suggested that, during development, a child's behavior is initially under the verbal control of others and only gradually does it come under the control of the child, first by overt speech and later by covert speech. According to this developmental model, during the first stage of the child's life the speech of others, typically the adults in their world, controls and directs his or her overt behavior. A child subsequently gains control over his or her own behavior through the use of overt self-instructions which, in the final stage, are ultimately internalized as covert self-instructions or inner speech.

Based on this model, a treatment paradigm was developed and used to teach children with impulsive behavior to talk to themselves (Meichenbaum & Goodman, 1971). Since their initial successful application, the procedures for teaching self-instructions have been replicated in numerous studies. Self-instruction training has also been successfully employed to decrease other types of behaviors such as aggression, hyperactivity, and fears, as well as to improve academic performance, and train social competence in children (e.g., Craighead, Wilcoxon-Craighead, & Meyers, 1978; Kratochwill & Morris, 1991; Mash & Barkley, 1989).

Components

The ultimate goal of self-instruction training is for children to internalize self-instructions so that they are able to use them in a variety of everyday situations. Since talking out loud to oneself is not considered a socially acceptable behavior in many situations, this typically means the instructor must teach the child to use the self-instructions covertly (i.e., silently). To do this, self-instructions are faded during training from overt (out loud) to whispering, and finally to covert (silent) speech. Specifically, the sequence of self-instruction training typically involves the following steps (Meichenbaum & Goodman, 1971):

1. *Cognitive modeling.* The instructor models appropriate behavior and talks out loud while the child observes. Verbalizations may be in the form of appraisals of task

requirements ("What do I have to do?"), guidance for performance ("I should try to read slowly and carefully"), statements of personal adequacy ("I'm good at this kind of problem"), statements to counteract worry over failure ("I know I can do this if I try hard"), and self-praise for successful performance ("Wow, I did a great job!").

2. *Overt external guidance.* The child performs the appropriate behavior while the instructor continues to talk out loud. The instructor verbally directs, guides, and praises the child's behavior.

3. *Overt self-guidance.* Now the child performs the appropriate behavior while talking out loud. The child rehearses verbalizations previously modeled by the instructor while engaging in the appropriate behavior.

4. *Faded overt self-guidance.* The child now performs the appropriate behavior while whispering the self-instructional statements.

5. *Covert self-instruction.* Finally, the child performs the appropriate behavior while (hopefully) engaging in covert self-instructions.

These steps are summarized in Table 4.2.

Over a number of training sessions, the self-statements initially modeled by the instructor and later rehearsed by the child are enlarged. For example, in the original Meichenbaum

TABLE 4.2. Self-Instruction Training Sequence

Instructor	Student
1. Self-talks out loud and performs task	1. Observes
2. Self-talks out loud	2. Performs task
3. Observes and prompts when necessary	3. Self-talks out loud and performs task
4. Observes and fades prompting	4. Whispers self-talk and performs task
5. Observes	5. Performs task silently

and Goodman (1971) study, the instructor performed a copying task while saying:

> "Okay, what is it I have to do? You want me to copy the picture with the different lines. I have to go slowly and carefully. Okay, draw the line down, down, good; and then to the right, that's it; now down some more and to the left. Good, I'm doing fine so far. Remember, go slowly. Now back up again. Now, I was supposed to go down. That's okay. Just erase the line carefully. . . . Good. Even if I make an error I can go on slowly and carefully. I have to go down now. Finished. I did it!" (p. 117)

In this example, the instructor demonstrated several skills including (1) problem definition ("What is it I have to do?"), (2) attention focusing and response guidance ("Carefully . . . Draw the line down"), (3) self-reinforcement ("Good, I'm doing fine"), and (4) self-evaluative coping skills and error correcting options ("That's okay . . . Even if I make an error I can go on slowly").

Outcome Studies

Self-instruction training has been applied to children of all ages who have a variety of problems. For example, self-instruction training has been used effectively to increase academic behaviors such as on-task and independent work performance (Bornstein & Quevillon, 1976; Bryant & Budd, 1982) and academic accuracy (Roberts et al., 1987; Swanson & Scarpati, 1985).

Despite these encouraging findings, self-instruction training has not always had positive results (e.g., Billings & Wasik, 1985; Friedling & O'Leary, 1979). In fact, results of one study suggest the effectiveness of self-instruction may be explained in terms of "setting" events. In other words, self-instruction training may simply provide the setting for "good clear instructions, reinforcement for memorizing those instructions, or reinforcement for accuracy in problem completion" (p. 241). Hence they are the important variables in the results obtained (Roberts et al., 1987). Continued research into the parameters of self-instruction training in school settings is still needed.

Implementation Considerations

There are a number of practical considerations that teachers must address prior to implementing self-instruction training. First, self-instruction training can be provided to an individual or to an entire group. With individual training, the instructor can be certain the child is focusing on critical steps in the process and can frequently check his or her grasp of the material being presented. However, the amount of time and effort required may not be justified, given that the instructor is impacting only one student. Group training is obviously more cost effective and potentially has a greater impact in that more students may benefit from the training. In addition, students may be exposed to peer modeling of self-talk behavior, which may enhance acquisition of this skill. However, with a group format, the instructor is less certain that individual students are actually acquiring the skills being presented. A compromise may be to involve a small group of students in training, and thereby maximize the potential impact on a limited number of students.

A second consideration involves the activity of self-talk. Since self-instruction typically is not a behavior that school-age children engage in naturally, warm-up exercises may be needed to familiarize students with the procedure and assist them in feeling comfortable with the idea of talking out loud to themselves. To do this, the instructor may begin the training by informally modeling self-talk with simple tasks. For example, while students watch, the instructor may use self-talk in preparing for the session:

"Let's see. What do I need for our session today? I need pencils, paper, and . . . Oh, I almost forgot! I need our math worksheets. I'll just go over to my desk and look in this pile. No, they're not here. Hum, where did I put them? . . . Oh, I remember, they're in the file cabinet. I'll just open the top drawer and look for the file folder labeled math worksheets.

Here they are! Good, I did it! Now I have everything. We have everything we need and we're ready to begin today's session . . ."

After discussing what they saw, the instructor may then assign each student a simple task that requires the completion of a series of steps, and then have the student use self-talk to direct his or her behavior. This not only helps the student who is engaging in the self-talk experience this procedure, but may also help other peers who are observing the process become accustomed to self-talk.

Third, the instructor must be prepared to have children involved in self-instruction training for an extended period of time. Typically, several training sessions are needed to teach students self-instruction skills. Even if students appear able to engage in self-talk after only a few sessions, they may not be comfortable with the idea of using this skill outside the training session for the reasons described above. In addition, since the goal is to teach students to use *covert* self-talk, repeated practice over an extended period of time using gradually reduced speech volume is essential to the success of the procedure.

It is also important to recognize that self-instruction is not appropriate for everyone. Some students never really accept nor enjoy using self-talk. These students may express discomfort at having to talk out loud in front of others and may be extremely resistant to any efforts to teach the procedure. Obviously with this procedure, and most other self-management interventions, student motivation to participate is essential. Highly resistant students are not good candidates for self-management interventions (see Chapter 5 for further discussion of student resistance).

Finally, a balance must be maintained between the requirements of the task itself and the self-instruction procedure. If too much emphasis is placed on self-instruction behavior, some children may actually become distracted and, as a result, their task performance may suffer. On the other hand, students should be encouraged to use self-instruction in several classroom, or other settings, to facilitate generalization of these skills across settings. Therefore, it is important to give careful consideration to the tasks to which self-instructions are to be applied. Initially, when students are just learning the self-instruction procedure, it is helpful to practice self-talk using very simple tasks or behaviors. Simple sensorimotor tasks such as copying line patterns and coloring figures within the boundaries given may be appropriate for young children, while relatively easy academic or interpersonal problems may be appropriate for older children and adolescents. However, once students are good at using self-instructions, it may be helpful to gradually increase the difficulty level of the tasks or situations provided. This allows students to practice using self-talk as a learning or problem-solving strategy and may facilitate their acquiring new concepts in a natural environment.

Case Example

A teacher designed a self-instruction strategy for three of her students who were having difficulty with addition and subtraction problems. Using a 12-inch ruler, she first constructed a number line that included the word "addition" with an arrow pointing to the right, and the word "subtraction" with an arrow pointing to the left. Using the Meichenbaum model for individual training sessions with students, the teacher initially modeled the self-talk while performing the desired behavior. Since none of these students had ever been exposed to self-talk, she introduced the procedure by demonstrating self-talk with simple actions (e.g., moving a pencil from one location to another) and having students imitate her behavior. Although two of the students required considerable prompting, all of them engaged in self-talk behavior by the end of the first session.

During the second session, each student was provided with the number line, a pencil, and a sheet containing addition or subtraction problems. The teacher introduced and modeled a 10-step procedure for completing addition or subtraction problems described in Table 4.3. For each problem, she stated:

"Let's see, what is my problem? I need to start with problem #1 here. I'm going to circle the '+' sign like this, so now

TABLE 4.3. Procedure for self-instruction in math

Materials: Marked number line
    Pencil
    Sheet of addition problems with sums up to 12

1. Ask "What is my problem?"
2. Circle "+" sign.
3. Match "+" sign to sign on number line.
4. Copy arrow over problem.
5. Find top/largest number on number line.
6. Hold place with finger or pencil.
7. Find bottom/smallest number and move in direction of arrow that many spaces on number line.
8. Read answer from number line.
9. Copy answer below equal sign.
10. Ask "How did I do?"

I know it's an addition problem. Now I'll go up to my number line and find that same '+' sign up here. There it is. And I see that the arrow goes this way. That means I need to move this way on the number line to solve this problem. Okay, I'll copy the arrow above Problem #1 to remind me which way to move on my number line . . Good. I did it right. Now, the largest number from this problem, 6 plus 3, is 6. And I'll find 6 on the number line . . . Here it is. I'll put my finger on the 6 while I look back at the problem. The other number is 3, so I need to move 3 spaces in the direction my arrow is pointing . . . 1 . . . 2 . . . 3. And the number I end on is 9. So the answer to this problem is 9. I'll write 9 here. How did I do? I did great!"

  Training proceeded in subsequent sessions with each student participating more, first by performing the behaviors while the teacher talked and later by performing the behaviors while engaging in self-talk. As students became more proficient at verbally guiding themselves through the 10-step procedure, they were instructed to talk more quietly until, during the last sessions, they were asked to whisper to themselves. All three students were able to learn the self-talk procedure and, as a result, made academic gains in mathematics. The teacher reported that the procedure was easy to implement and she would consider using it again in the future. Students reported that they enjoyed using the number lines and engaging in the self-talk procedures.

STRESS-INOCULATION TRAINING

Description

The second major category of cognitive-based interventions, termed coping-skills approaches, includes procedures designed to teach individuals more adaptive methods of coping with stress-producing situations. One example of this type of intervention is stress-inoculation training. Stress-inoculation training is a cognitive-based self-management intervention designed to treat anger and anxiety problems. The primary goal is to develop the child's competence to adapt to stressful events in such a way that stress is manageable and the child able to function more productively in his or her environment. A primary focus is on learning to cope with stress rather than completely eliminating it from the child's life. The rationale is that children will regularly encounter, as part of their daily existence, events that produce feelings of anger or anxiety. This is a part of life and something that none of us can control completely. As such, it is reasoned that the most beneficial approach for children with excessive anger or anxiety reactions may be to teach them specific ways to cope with these regularly occurring stressors. Hence, the procedure integrates training in both cognitive and relaxation skills to promote adaptive coping with stress or provocation. Although it is obvious that academic difficulties would not be the primary target of stress-inoculation training, it is conceivable that a child may be experiencing severe stress in response to academic task demands.

Background

As with self-instruction training, Meichenbaum (1972, 1977) is primarily responsible for delineating stress-inoculation training procedures. The term "inoculation" functions as a medical metaphor to express the process whereby the child is gradually exposed to manageable doses of a stressor and, in this way, is prepared to cope with the stressful event when it actually occurs in the natural environment (Novaco, 1978). Characteristic of cognitive-based approaches, the child's maladaptive anger or anxiety response is viewed as a result of both heightened emotional arousal and faulty cognitions. In other words, emotional arousal, and the child's subsequent behavior, are thought to be determined by how the child perceives the situation. For example, a child who is emotionally aroused (i.e., anxious) during an oral presentation to the class is more likely to perform the activity appropriately if she views the event as "fun." However, the same student may perform poorly during a similar oral presentation if the situation is perceived as being negative.

Components

Stress-inoculation training targets both emotional arousal (anger or anxiety) and cognitions (thoughts). The relaxation component of stress-inoculation is designed to reduce heightened arousal and the cognitive restructuring component, which includes a form of self-instruction training, is intended to reduce dysfunctional cognitions. Training in the use of the stress-inoculation approach typically involves three basic steps or phases: cognitive preparation, skill acquisition, and application practice. These are summarized in Table 4.4.

TABLE 4.4. Stress-Inoculation Training

Phases	Activities
Cognitive preparation	Presentation of conceptual framework Discussion of diary Identification of anger/anxiety cues
Skill acquisition	Cognitive restructuring training Self-instruction training Relaxation training
Application practice	Rehearsal of new coping skills

Cognitive Preparation

The cognitive preparation phase is designed to educate the child about the functions of anger or anxiety and to introduce the rationale for treatment. The child is given a conceptual framework, in age-appropriate language, to assist in understanding the nature of his or her specific responses to stressful events. The child is also asked to keep a diary, which serves as a basis of discussion of specific personal anger/anxiety patterns. Examples of the topics discussed during the cognitive preparation phase include (Novaco, 1978):

1. *Identifying persons and situations that trigger anger or anxiety.* Information from the child's diary is often helpful in pinpointing those events that will most likely produce excessive anger or anxiety reactions in this particular child.
2. *Distinguishing anger or anxiety from aggression.* As these are frequently children who engage in aggressive behavior, it is important to make the distinction between the expression of appropriate and inappropriate feelings. This also introduces the notion that we have a choice as to how we are going to react to situations and express the feelings we have.
3. *Discriminating justified from less justified anger or anxiety.* Individual events/situations are examined carefully in an effort to make this distinction.
4. *Understanding the cues for anger or anxiety.* The child is taught to identify specific "buttons" that, if pushed, may cause him or her to become angry or anxious.
5. *Understanding anger or anxiety in terms of interaction sequences.* Behavior is viewed in terms of the child's social context rather than as something that occurs in isolation.
6. *Introducing anger or anxiety management techniques as coping strategies to handle conflict and stress.* Handling stressful situations in an appropriate, competent manner is portrayed as a set of skills that can be taught and learned.

Skill Acquisition

Training in the areas of cognitive restructuring and relaxation is provided during this phase using modeling and behavior rehearsal techniques. The child is provided with a variety of specific coping techniques to use in potentially stressful situations in an effort to prevent maladaptive anger or anxiety reactions. At the cognitive level, the child is taught to view specific stressful events differently (e.g., reduce the exaggerated importance often attached to stressful events). Special emphasis is placed on learning to "not take things personally" and on maintaining a sense of humor. The primary goal of cognitive restructuring is to promote flexibility in the way the child views stressful situations. An important aspect of this restructuring is the use of self-instructions (Meichenbaum, 1977). As discussed in the previous section, self-instructions serve as instructional cues that guide the child's thoughts, feelings, and behavior (Novaco, 1978). These cognitive strategies are used in combination with Jacobson's (1938) relaxation training procedures, which involves systematically tensing and relaxing various muscle groups in an effort to teach relaxation as an alternative physiological response to stressful situations.

Application Practice

The third and final phase of stress-inoculation training is termed application practice. Activities in this phase involve testing the child's ability to manage stressful situations. Typically, the instructor uses imagery and role playing to induce the emotional arousal (anger or anxiety), while the child practices the newly acquired coping responses (self-statements and relaxation). Thus, in response to the emotional arousal, the child activates the relaxation coping skills to reduce arousal and the cognitive self-instructions to change faulty cognitive mediation of anger/anxiety (Deffenbacher & Suinn, 1982). More specifically, a hierarchy of anger or anxiety situations from most intense to least arousing is constructed with the child. Beginning with the least arousing, the instructor simulates each situation while the child practices the newly acquired cognitive and relaxation skills. When the child masters dealing with that situation, increasingly provocative scenes are introduced until the child is able to imagine or role play the most intense situations while engaging in coping behaviors. The child is also instructed to apply his or her newly acquired skills to controlling anger or anxiety between formal sessions in the natural environment to facilitate transfer of skills from training to real-life situations.

Outcome Studies

Stress-inoculation has been shown to be an effective treatment for a variety of targeted problems. In an early study, Meichenbaum (1972) found stress-inoculation to be as effective as, and in some cases more effective than, a systematic desensitization procedure for reducing text anxiety. Other successfully treated problems include anger (Novaco, 1977b), depression (Novaco, 1977a), speech anxiety (Fremouw & Zitter, 1978), and lack of assertiveness (Safran, Alden, & Davidson, 1980). Stress-inoculation has also been used frequently with children in the successful treatment of stress associated with medical and dental procedures (Peterson & Shigetomi, 1981; Siegel & Peterson, 1980).

Implementation Considerations

As stress-inoculation training involves a number of cognitive and relaxation strategies, its usefulness is limited to those children who have the cognitive skills to understand, acquire, and use these procedures. At a minimum, this would involve an ability to achieve a state of relaxation, imagine and role play stressful situations, and employ covert self-statements. Thus, stress-inoculation is appropriate for older children and adolescents who are experiencing excessive or maladaptive anger or anxiety in response to specific situations they encounter regularly in the school environment. Examples of common stressful situations include test anxiety, anxiety around public speaking, and excessive anger in response to interpersonal situations. Stress-inoculation is not appropriate for use with young children or students with moderate or more severe cognitive disabilities.

Providing a student with stress-inoculation training is a time consuming endeavor and, due to the nature of the procedure, typically involves individual training. Because the strategy is time consuming and costly to implement, it probably should be limited to only the most severe anger or anxiety management problems. The procedure could conceivably be modified for a small group of students with similar problems (e.g., anger control), although no examples of this can be found in the literature. To do this effectively with a small group of students, it may be necessary to adopt a social skills training format (described in a subsequent section) and rely more on role playing than on cognitive imagery.

Case Example

A fifth-grade student named Erica was referred by her teacher to the school's prereferral intervention team for consultation regarding her severe anxiety reactions, which apparently surrounded testing situations. The team learned from the teacher that the problem had progressed to the point that Erica actually became physically ill immediately preceding a test. The team also learned that Erica's academic performance in most areas was average, although deficits had been noted in mathematics. This was consistent with teacher reports that the most serious reactions preceded tests in math, although these reactions also occurred now prior to tests in English and science.

Interviews with Erica confirmed an intense fear of failure in most academic areas, especially math. She reported feeling nauseated, tense, sweaty, and short of breath prior to a scheduled exam. As this problem appeared to be directly related to anxiety surrounding math performance, the team recommended individual tutoring in math and stress inoculation training to be conducted by the school psychologist.

The school psychologist met individually with Erica for 45 minutes, twice a week, for a period of 20 weeks. During the initial 4-week cognitive preparation phase of training, objectives were (1) to establish a collaborative relationship, (2) to collect information in the form of interviews, questionnaires, self-monitoring procedures, imagery-based techniques, and behavioral assessments, and (3) to establish goals for training. The information-gathering activities were designed to provide specific examples of stressful events and resulting reactions, and to increase Erica's awareness of her contribution to these reactions. Imagery-based recall (Meichenbaum, 1985) was one useful means of helping Erica report specific information that otherwise may have been overlooked or underemphasized in a direct interview. Using this procedure, the school psychologist asked Erica to imagine one (or several) recent stress experiences. She was then asked to recall the experience as clearly as possible and visualize it as if she were there at that moment:

"Okay, Erica, we're going to try something different today that may give us more information about your reaction to tests. I'd like you to think about one stressful testing experience that you had recently, and I want you to try to visualize it as if you are actually there now. Can you think of one? Okay, good. Just sit back in your chair, close your eyes, and think about the experience. Take your time, there's no rush. Begin at the point just before you felt any real stress. Then replay the entire event in your imagination in slow motion. Talk to me as you go. Tell me anything you remember seeing, thinking, feeling, or doing."

Erica also self-monitored her reactions to each stressful experience by recording what happened immediately before she began to feel stressed; her thoughts, feelings, and behavior during each stress episode; and what happened immediately after the episode. In addition, she was also asked to keep a diary of her general moods and any insights that she might have related to this problem. Throughout this initial phase of training, the school psychologist reinforced the concept that ultimately Erica had control over the stress reaction, and created a positive expectancy that the problem would be solved.

The 8-week skill acquisition phase of training was designed to teach Erica specific relaxation skills and cognitive strategies to use in testing situations. Although there are several different procedures available to teach relaxation skills, the school psychologist decided to design a relaxation training procedure for Erica based on the techniques developed by Jacobson (1938). Using this method, Erica was taught to discriminate alternate states of tension and relaxation as they were applied sequentially to various muscle groups. The school psychologist asked Erica to lean back in her chair and close her eyes, and then stated:

"I am going to teach you how to become very relaxed. In doing this, I am going to ask you to tense and relax different sets of muscles so that you become more and more relaxed throughout your whole body. Clear your mind of any distracting thoughts . . . Okay, now I am going to focus your attention on various muscle groups. Whenever I say the word 'tense,' I would like you to take a deep breath and tense that particular muscle group until I say 'relax.' Remember, keep that muscle group tensed and hold your breath until I say 'relax.' Let's begin by focusing on your right hand. Breath normally. When I say the word 'tense,' I want you to take a deep breath and tense all the muscles in your right fist. Hold it until I say 'relax.' Any questions? Okay. Focus on your right hand. Ready . . . tense. Hold it, hold it. Feel the tension in that hand. Harder . . . Okay, relax. Let all the air out of your lungs. Let all the tension flow out of your hand. Just relax and breathe normally. Notice the feeling of relaxation . . . Good, now let's shift the focus to your left hand. . . . "

Relaxation training proceeded in this manner until all major muscle groups were targeted and Erica indicated she was in a relaxed state. As training progressed, the number of muscle groups targeted was decreased and Erica was encouraged to use the cue words, "tense" and "relax" herself. Erica was also encouraged to practice achieving a state of relaxation several times during the day outside of the training setting.

A number of cognitive procedures were used in an effort to modify Erica's thoughts and feelings about testing situations. These included cognitive restructuring, problem solving, and self-instruction. The cognitive restructuring component was designed to make Erica aware of the role cognitions and emotions played in initiating and maintaining her stress. The main techniques of the cognitive restructuring approach used with Erica were based on Beck's work on cognitive therapy, and included (Beck, Rush, Hollon, & Shaw, 1979):

1. Eliciting Erica's thoughts, feelings, and interpretation of stressful events.
2. Gathering evidence with Erica for or against these interpretations.
3. Setting up situations to test the validity of the interpretations and to gather more data for discussion.

As an example of the first item in the list, one activity was designed to assist Erica in identifying specific random thoughts she may be having about the testing experience, termed *automatic thoughts* (Beck, 1963). The purpose of this exercise was to help Erica recognize that many of her negative thoughts were inferences, not facts as she assumed them to be. Some of the automatic thoughts reported by Erica included, "I'll never be any good at math," "I'm the only one who doesn't understand this stuff," and "There's nothing I can do to pass this test." The school psychologist then asked Erica for evidence that these automatic thoughts were actually valid.

Both problem-solving training (discussed in the subsequent section) and self-instruction training (described in the previous section) were used by having Erica ask herself a series of questions prior to each testing situation. These included the following (Wasik, 1984):

1. Problem identification: "What is the concern?"
2. Goal selection: "What do I want?"
3. Generation of alternatives: "What can I do?"
4. Consideration of consequences: "What might happen?"
5. Decision making: "What is my decision?"
6. Implementation: "Now do it!"
7. Evaluation: "Did it work?"

During the final 8 weeks of training, specific stress-producing situations were simulated to provide Erica with an opportunity to practice the relaxation skills and cognitive strategies she had learned during the previous 8 weeks. The focus was primarily on testing situations that Erica would be encountering in the near future. Imagery procedures similar to those described previously were used to help Erica visualize each experience and her appropriate coping reactions to it. During the last 2 weeks of training, exercises included actually walking to the hallway outside the classroom in which Erica would be taking a test and having Erica verbally rehearse the procedures she had learned there.

Using this combination of strategies and working closely with the math tutor to ensure her success, the school psychologist reported significant gains in Erica's cognitive and relaxation skills. In addition, the teacher reported a dramatic improvement in Erica's test behavior and test scores, as she achieved a passing grade on all the math tests she took during the final half of school year. From Erica's perspective, she reported feeling much better about herself and more competent in a variety of academic areas including mathematics.

PROBLEM-SOLVING TRAINING

Description

The third major type of cognitive-based self-management intervention involves a problem-solving approach to emotional and behavior difficulties in children. In this case, inappropriate behavior is presumed to reflect a child's deficits in appropriate thinking or social skills. For example, a child who strikes out when teased by a peer may not know how else to handle the situation, never having learned a more appropriate response. Intervention based on this hypothesis may involve systematically identifying and teaching the child more appropriate social responses to potential conflict situations. The goal of these interventions is for the child to develop thinking or social skills that will enhance his or her adaptive behavior. As with other cognitive-based approaches, the skills taught are designed to influence what children are thinking and feeling in an effort to change their overt actions.

The classic definition of problem solving, as expressed by D'Zurilla and Goldfried (1971), is "a behavioral process . . . which (a) makes available a variety of potentially effective response alternatives for dealing with the problematic situation and (b) increases the probability of selecting the most effective response from among these various alternatives" (p. 108). Despite some similarities between problem solving and self-instruction, there are important differences that should be noted. Although self-instruction training has a problem-solving focus, many problem-solving strategies do not emphasize self-statements (Kendall & Braswell, 1985). In addition, the scope of social problem-solving training is generally more extensive than that of self-instruction training (Keogh & Hall, 1984).

Background

Problem-solving originally developed from the cognitive psychology literature and was introduced into behavior therapy in 1971 by D'Zurilla and Goldfried. Based on the general problem-solving literature, these writers suggested a five-stage model of problem solving, which is summarized in Table 4.5. A number of investigations provided evidence that children with various disabilities were indeed deficient or inconsistent in the generation and use of appropriate problem-solving strategies, including children with learning disabilities (Keogh & Hall, 1984), mental retardation (Miller, Hale, & Stevenson, 1968), and impulsivity and aggression (Spivack & Shure, 1974; Spivack, Platt, & Shure, 1976). One of the first successful applications of D'Zurilla and Goldfried's (1971) model with children was Spivack and Shure's (1974) work on the assessment and training of problem-solving skills in aggressive and impulsive children. Subsequently, a number of problem-solving and social skills training programs were developed, all designed to teach children a variety of strategies for improving interper-

TABLE 4.5. D'Zurilla and Goldfried's Problem-Solving Model

Step	Description of activities
1. General orientation	Provide a "set" so that child perceives interpersonal interactions as problems to be solved.
2. Problem definition and formulation	Define and operationalize specific problem situations.
3. Generation of alternatives	Generate a large number of possible solutions to specific problems.
4. Decision making	Estimate the probable consequences of the alternative responses (from #3) and choose the most favorable alternative.
5. Verification	Evaluate the outcome of the response chosen. If not satisfactory, return to earlier steps.

sonal relationships, managing anger, or developing positive cognitions.

Components

As there is no one generally accepted model for social problem solving, several examples are provided here. Three popular approaches are "I Can Problem Solve" (Shure, 1992a, 1992b, 1992c), "Think Aloud" (Camp & Bash, 1985a, 1985b, 1985c), and the "Skill-streaming" programs (Goldstein et al., 1980; McGinnis & Goldstein, 1992, 1984).

The "I Can Problem Solve" Program

In the recently published "I Can Problem Solve" (ICPS) manuals for preschool, kindergarten/primary grades, and intermediate elementary grades, Shure (1992a, 1992b, 1992c) presents a cognitive problem-solving program that is the result of over 20 years of research and development by a group of researchers at Hahnemann University. Early research with adolescents demonstrated a clear association between interpersonal cognitive problem-solving skills and behavior. This early work was designed to enhance interpersonal thinking skills to prevent or reduce high-risk behaviors (Spivack et al., 1976). The underlying goal of the current program continues to be "to help children learn *how* to think, not *what* to think" (p. 1). Rather than providing them with specific suggestions for what to do in conflict or problem situations, the program offers children ways to think through problems. The program has been field tested in urban and suburban school districts throughout the country. The main goal, focus, content, methods, and benefits of ICPS are summarized in Table 4.6.

The ICPS manuals include formal lessons as well as specific suggestions for incorporating problem-solving strategies into classroom interactions/curriculum. Each lesson includes (1) a stated purpose, (2) suggested materials, and (3) a teacher script. As described in the manuals, the teacher script is intended to be a flexible guideline for implementing the basic steps of the lesson. Lessons are grouped into two major categories: pre-problem-solving skills and problem-solving skills. Pre-problem-solving concepts set the stage for the acquisition of problem-solving skills by teaching the ICPS vocabulary (e.g., IS–NOT, IF–THEN, SAME–DIFFERENT), helping children identify feelings (e.g., happy, sad, angry), and by encouraging listening and paying attention skills. Problem-solving skills involve the concepts of (1) alternative solutions, (2) consequences, and (3) solution-consequence pairs. Alternative-solutions lessons are designed to help children recognize problems and generate possible solutions. The objective of consequences sessions is to help children learn to think sequentially and engage in consequential thinking. Finally, solution–consequence pair lessons are designed to give children practice in linking solutions with consequences. Although Shure (1992a, 1992b, 1992c) notes it is possible to conduct ICPS lessons with an entire class of 30 children, she suggests smaller groups may be preferable to increase the opportunities for each child to participate. It is estimated that, if daily 20- to 40-minute lessons are conducted, it will take approximately 4 months to complete the program.

TABLE 4.6. The "I Can Problem Solve" Program

GOAL	To teach children thinking skills that can be used to help resolve or prevent "people" problems
FOCUS	Teaches children *how* to think, not *what* to think Guides children to think for themselves Teaches children how to evaluate their own ideas Encourages children to come up with many solutions to problems on their own
CONTENT	*Pre-problem-solving skills* Learning a problem-solving vocabulary Identifying one's own and others' feelings Considering other people's points of view *Problem-solving skills* Thinking of more than one solution Considering consequences Deciding which solution to choose
METHOD	Teaches skills through the use of games, stories, puppets, and role-playing Guides the use of skills in real-life situations
BENEFITS	*For children* Fun for children, presents lessons in game form Builds self-confidence Encourages generation of alternative solutions Provides skills to handle new problems Facilitates social interaction among peers Teaches skills applicable to other situations Increases sensitivity to others Increases independence *For teachers* Reinforces other curriculum goals Creates a more positive classroom atmosphere Decreases time spent in handling conflicts Uses "pyramid" learning (in other words, lessons build on one another) Teaches skills applicable to other situations Enhances teachers' own problem-solving skills

Note. From *I Can Problem Solve* (p. 2) by M. B. Shure, 1992, Champaign, IL: Research Press. Copyright 1992 by Myrna B. Shure. Reprinted by permission.

Teacher creativity with the content is encouraged and role playing is recommended for those children who can engage in that activity as both a practice and a motivational technique.

An example of one lesson from the ICPS manual for kindergarten and the primary grades (Shure, 1992b) is provided here. This lesson is from the problem-solving skills section of the manual and is entitled, "What Else Can He Do?" (Part I, Lesson 48). The lesson is designed to encourage children to think of as many solutions to a problem as they can. Materials required include an illustration of a boy and his mother in a grocery store (see Figure 4.1) and a chalkboard or easel. The teacher begins by showing the children the illustration and saying:

> "The problem in this picture is that this boy (*point*) wants his mother to buy him this box of cookies. What does the boy want his mother to do? Right, buy him the box of cookies.
>
> Now we're going to play the What Else Can He Do Game. We want to think of lots of ways, lots of DIFFERENT solutions to this problem. I'm going to write ALL your ideas to solve the problem on the chalkboard. Who's got way number one? (*Show one finger.*)" (p. 227)

The teacher records relevant responses verbatim (e.g., "He could ask her"), asks for clarification for unclear responses (e.g., "He could cry" may be followed with a prompt to "Tell me more about that"), and states, "How would that help solve the problem?" for irrelevant responses. Teachers are reminded to provide specific praise for *different* solutions (i.e., rather than saying, "That's a good idea, " state, "Good, that's a DIFFERENT idea"). Significantly, the latter will tend to promote a broader variety of solutions, whereas the former may encourage enumerations of the same basic idea. At the end of the session the teacher summarizes all the solutions written on the board. A similar format is followed in each ICPS lesson. For more detailed information concerning the ICPS program, interested readers may wish to consult the recently published manuals (Shure, 1992a, 1992b, 1992c).

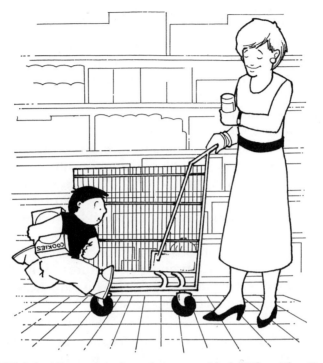

FIGURE 4.1. Illustration from lesson entitled "What Else Can He Do?" (Part I). From *I can Problem Solve: An Interpersonal Cognitive Problem-Solving Program (Kindergarten and Primary Grades)* (p. 231) by M. B. Shure, 1992b. Copyright 1992 by Myrna B. Shure. Reprinted by permission.

The "Think Aloud" Program

Another popular problem-solving training program for use in classroom settings is the "Think Aloud" program, which was first developed by Camp et al. (1977). This program was designed as a psychoeducational training program that could be carried out by teachers for the purpose of enhancing self-control in aggressive students. The "Think Aloud" program guides (Camp & Bash, 1985a, 1985b, 1985c) include detailed lesson plans, and specific materials and dialogues that cover approximately 40 sessions.

The lessons begin with the use of "Copy Cat" activities designed to ensure that children imitate both the words and actions of their teacher. During these activities, the teacher makes simple statements (e.g., "I'm supposed to color this circle") and gestures (e.g., coloring the circle), which the children are prompted to repeat.

In subsequent lessons, children play "Copy Cat" while the teacher models ways of thinking through a problem and coping with mistakes. Using cognitive problems such as puzzles, mazes, and matrices, students are taught to answer four basic questions: "What is my problem?", "What is my plan?", "Am I using my plan?", and "How did I do?" Cue pictures, illustrated in Figure 4.2, are introduced to help children remember and use these questions.

Finally, social problems are introduced using a combination of problem-solving training procedures (Spivack et al., 1976) and self-instructional strategies. This sequence of lessons moves through the following stages:

1. Identifying and expressing feelings, and the basic language of cause and effect (e.g., why–because, if–then, what might happen next).
2. Generating alternative solutions to social problems.
3. Generating possible consequences of actions.
4. Developing evaluation skills.
5. For specific problems, developing solutions and potential consequences, and evaluating each.

Thus, the program is designed to move from learning the relatively simple skills of imitating words and actions, and using questions to organize one's approach to problem solving, to the more complex skills of generating alternative solutions, verbalizing plans independently, and self-monitoring and self-evaluating actions. In addition, students are given increasingly difficult problems, which involve following complex directions using negative commands or which require independent thinking, typically at some physical distance from the teacher. For more detailed information concerning the "Think Aloud"

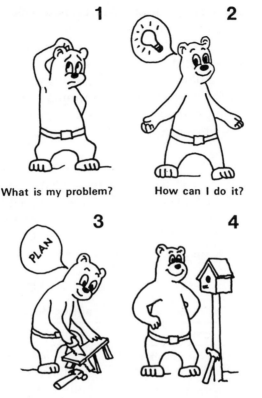

FIGURE 4.2. Cue pictures used in the "Think Aloud" program. From *Think Aloud: Increasing Social and Cognitive Skills* A problem-solving program for children; grades 1–2 (p. 56) by B. W. Camp & S. M Bash, 1985, Champaign, IL: Research Press. Copyright 1985 by Research Press. Reprinted by permission.

program, interested readers may wish to consult the "Think Aloud" program guides (Camp & Bash, 1985a, 1985b, 1985c).

Social Skills Training

One example of a social skills training program for use with children and adolescents in classroom settings is Goldstein and colleagues' multicomponent problem-solving training program (Goldstein et al., 1980; McGinnis & Goldstein, 1984, 1992). The program was originally designed for use with groups of aggressive adolescents and then was expanded to include preschool- and elementary-aged students with a variety of difficulties. This structured learning approach consists of a number of therapy procedures recommended by Bandura (1973), including verbal instruction, modeling, role playing, performance feedback, and transfer of training. These procedures are summarized in Table 4.7.

With the *verbal instruction* procedure, the skill to be taught during that session is described to students, as well as the situations in which it may be useful to them. Specific behavioral steps that constitute that skill are presented verbally, and on a chalkboard or easel. Although this represents but a brief introduction, it is important in that it sets the stage for the

TABLE 4.7. Social Skills Training Procedures

Procedure	Description	Purpose
Verbal instruction	Description of specific skill to be taught	Creates a cognitive set; stimulates student interest and motivation
Modeling	Live vignettes by instructors enacting the skill being taught	Provides a clear display of the specific behavioral steps that constitute this skill
Role playing	Behavioral rehearsal or practice by students	Provides opportunities to practice behavioral steps the instructor modeled; enhances future use of the skill
Feedback	Specific corrective feedback and praise	Provides information on how well behavioral steps were followed; increases motivation to use the skill in real life
Transfer of learning	Homework assignments, external support, and self-reward	Increases the likelihood learning will transfer to real-life situations

remainder of the session, and stimulates student interest and motivation for participation.

Next, instructors move to *modeling* the skill being taught. Here, the instructors portray the specific behavioral steps of the skill in a variety of settings relevant to the students' daily lives. Students' attention is directed to how the actors in each vignette model the specific behavioral steps. *Role playing* is used to encourage realistic behavioral rehearsal by children. To enhance realism, the primary actor is asked to choose a peer to play the role of another person who is relevant to the skills problem. Children are encouraged to engage in the specific behavioral steps while role playing.

Upon completion of each role play, brief *performance feedback* is provided. This consists of such information as how well the trainees followed the steps, in what ways they departed from them, the potential impact of their behaviors on others, and encouragement to use the behaviors that were role played in real life. Finally, *transfer-of-training* procedures are used to enhance the transfer and the maintenance of the skills learned during training to the real life settings of the students. These procedures include assigning homework, enlisting the support of individuals in the students' school or home environments, and teaching self-management strategies such as self-monitoring and self-reinforcement.

Separate manuals have been published for use with early childhood populations (McGinnis & Goldstein, 1992), elementary-aged students (McGinnis & Goldstein, 1984), and adolescents (Goldstein et al., 1980). Each manual includes information concerning the general components of the program, assessment for selection and grouping of students, beginning and conducting a training group, as well as specific training content. Each prosocial skill to be taught includes identification of the steps involved in performing the skill, suggestions for specific points that should be discussed regarding each of these steps, common situations involving the skill, and additional comments. The manuals also provide transcripts of training sessions and suggestions for implementing the program, particularly with students who exhibit behavior problems.

Staying out of fights is an example of a skill alternative to aggression taught to elementary-aged children. As described in Table 4.8, several behavioral steps are identified for the development of this skill. Using verbal instruction, students are taught, modeling, role playing, and performance feedback, to approach potential problem situations such as peer teasing by engaging in the specific steps listed in Table 4.8 (i.e., stop and count to 10, decide what the problem is, think about the choices, and act out the best choice). The manual suggests that students in the upper elementary grades will guide the

TABLE 4.8. Skill Alternatives to Aggression: Staying Out of Fights

Steps	Notes for discussion
1. Stop and count to 10	Discuss how this step can help the student to calm down
2. Decide what the problem is	Discuss the consequences of fighting and whether fighting can solve the problem
3. Think about your choices:	List a variety of alternatives
• Walk away for now	Student should ask to leave the room for a few minutes, if necessary
• Talk to the person in a friendly way	Discuss how to read the behavior of the other person (i.e., is he/she calm enough to talk with) and evaluate the students own degree of calmness and readiness to talk about the problem; discuss ways to state the problem in a nonoffensive manner
• Ask someone for help in solving the problem	Discuss who can be of the most help: a teacher, parent, or friend
4. Act out your best choice	If one choice doesn't work, the student should try another one

Note. The following are possible situations to apply the steps to: *School*—Someone says that you did poorly on your schoolwork; *Home*—Your brother or sister tattles on you; *Peer group*—Someone doesn't play fairly in a game or calls you a name.

Adapted from *Skillstreaming the Elementary School Child: A Guide for Teaching Prosocial Skills*, by E. McGinnis & A. P. Goldstein with R. P. Sprafkin, & N. J. Gershaw, 1984, Champain, IL: Research Press. Copyright 1984 by E. McGinnis, A. P. Goldstein, R. P. Sprafkin, & N. J. Gershaw. Reprinted by permission.

group leaders to the level of complexity in these steps that they are able to handle, and that it may be necessary to simplify many steps for the effective instruction of children in the primary grades. Teaching a skill such as staying out of fights may require several sessions, especially for young elementary-aged children.

Outcome Studies

Reviews of the social skills and social problem-solving literature with children generally have reported positive results (e.g., Ager & Cole, 1991; Goldstein & Pentz, 1984; Gresham, 1985). For example, several controlled studies have been conducted to evaluate the "Think Aloud" program with young, aggressive boys. Each study included, at a minimum, measures of cognitive change and teacher ratings of classroom behavior. In addition, some investigations also included direct behavior observations by an independent observer. The program was revised over time to strengthen the social problem-solving component which involved having boys work together in pairs during each lesson. Each investigation revealed positive changes had occured in the behavior of the boys and teacher perceptions, indicating the value of this type of multicomponent program for the treatment of aggressive behavior in young boys (Camp, 1980; Camp & Bash, 1981; Camp et al., 1977).

In a review of 30 studies of social skills training with aggressive adolescents, Goldstein and Pentz (1984) concluded that the results for skills acquisition have been consistently positive. Aggressive adolescents are able to learn a variety of new interpersonal, aggressive-management, affect-relevant, and related psychological skills by using this skills training approach. However, the maintenance and transfer of these newly acquired skills appears to occur only when training procedures explicitly designed to enhance generalization are implemented. Other reviews have generally confirmed this finding (Ager & Cole, 1991; Gresham, 1985). However, a few recent studies reported promising evidence of enhanced maintenance and generalization with procedures involving the training of parents, using actual setting events to develop interventions, and employing additional self-management components (e.g., Knapczyk, 19i8; Lochman & Curry, 1986; Serna, Schumaker, Hazel, & Sheldon, 1986).

Implementation Considerations

Length of social problem-solving training in examples found in the literature range from a single 10-minute training session per child (Zahavi & Asher, 1978) to daily 20- to 40-minute sessions for 4 months (Shure, 1992a, 1992b, 1992c). It is certainly typical for social problem-solving training programs to involve daily individual or small group sessions extending over a period of several months. Obviously, significant changes in complex problem behavior cannot be expected to occur overnight. Approaches such as the ones described here require a considerable investment of time and resources if they are to produce durable and generalizable behavior change in students with difficulties. As noted by Shure (1992a, 1992b, 1992c), it may take 2 or 3 months for some inhibited children to begin participating, and even longer for actual changes in impulsive behavior to occur.

Since social problem-solving training typically involves a great deal of child participation, the composition of the group is important. It would be unwise, for example, to select only those children who are shy and nonresponsive for training. A better combination may be to involve both responders, to serve as role models, and nonresponders, who may need training the most, in a social problem-solving group. Another consideration in grouping children is what to do with children who are particularly disruptive. Again, placing all disruptive children in one group may be disastrous. Shure (1992a, 1992b, 1992c) also suggests separating disruptive children who are friends from each other.

As with many group training programs, it is helpful to have a teacher aide to assist with the training. This person could perform a variety of useful activities, including quietly prompting children to respond, assisting with disruptive students, or working with those students who are not involved in the formal training. In another scenario, the teacher aide could conduct formal training sessions with one half of the class, as the teacher is working with the other half. At a minimum, it is important that the teacher aide be familiar with the concepts being taught so that these can be reinforced outside formal training sessions during all school-day activities.

Case Example

A group of four sixth-grade students identified by the teacher as being the most disruptive students in her class were selected for social skills training. Assessment activities that resulted in the selection of these students included completion of (1) a daily log over a 2-week period, indicating antecedents and consequences of problem behaviors during time periods in which problems were likely to occur, and (2) the Social Skills Rating Scale (SSRS, Gresham & Elliott, 1990). The SSRS is a standardized assessment tool designed to identify specific social skills deficits in children.

Students are provided with social skills training for 30 minutes a day, 3 days a week. Skills corresponding to those identified during assessment are targeted for intervention. For example, one of the skills considered to be a priority by the teacher and identified as a deficit on the SSRS is *responding to teasing*. During the session, the teacher introduces this skill by stating:

"Today we're going to talk about how to respond to teasing. An example of this type of situation is when another student teases you or calls you names. Teasing from others is a normal part of everyday life, but it is important that you have the skills for responding to teasing appropriately. This way you can stay out of trouble and maybe even prevent the person from teasing you again."

The teacher chooses to use the "Skillstreaming" program (McGinnis & Goldstein, 1984) in providing the social problem-solving training. As indicated in the manual in the section termed Skill 38, the specific steps involved in the skill of responding to teasing include:

1. Stop and count to five.
2. Think about your choices:
   a. Ignore the teasing.
   b. Say how you feel, in a friendly way.
   c. Give a reason for the person to stop.
3. Act out your best choice.

These steps are written on the chalkboard prior to the session. The teacher reviews each of these briefly and then states, "Now watch closely how this student responds to teasing by another boy in his class."

The teacher and co-instructor then model a scenario in which a child is pushed and teased by someone in the cafeteria at lunch. The target "student" initially becomes angry but catches himself and begins the problem-solving process outlined on the chalkboard:

"I feel myself getting upset . . . I'm going to count to five . . . one, two, three, four, five. What choices do I have? I could just ignore him and walk away, but the other kids are looking and they might think I'm a sissy if I do that. I could say something like, 'Don't push me, and I don't like your teasing either.' That'd be okay I guess. Or I could give him a reason to stop like, 'You'd better stop that or we're both going to get in trouble.' I think I'll try the second one . . . 'Hey, stop pushing and teasing me. I don't like that' . . . Hey, I think it worked. He's walking away. I did it! That makes me feel good!"

Following the role play, the teacher asks for specific feedback from each student in the group: "What did you like about what he did?" or "What did he do correctly?" Then the teacher asks for feedback on how well the "student" implemented the specific steps of the skill: "Did he stop and count to five?" "How did he do with ignoring the teasing?" Finally, students are asked, "What could he do better next time?"

During the last half of the session, each student is provided with an opportunity to rehearse the behavioral steps involved in responding to a simulated teasing situation. Student input is solicited in creating a scenario that is relevant for him or her (e.g., an incident that occurred recently or that the student anticipates may occur in the near future). The teacher or co-instructor plays the role of the other person involved in each situation and is the first to respond during the feedback activity. An excerpt delineating this type of performance feedback is provided:

TEACHER 1: Mr. Adler, how do you feel about what Jason said?

TEACHER 2: I respected what he had to say. His voice volume was good and he was very polite in his response to my teasing. I think his message would have been more effective though if he had maintained eye contact when talking with me. I got the feeling he was a little uncomfortable.

TEACHER 1: Thanks, Mr. Adler. Okay, did Jason follow Step 1, Mike?

MIKE: Yeah.

TEACHER 1: What did he do?

MIKE: He counted to 10.

TEACHER 1: Yes, he did. Good. Did Jason follow Step 2a, Chuck?

CHUCK: Um, I guess so.

TEACHER 1: What makes you think he did that step?

CHUCK: Well, he didn't punch him out. He just ignored the teasing.

TEACHER 1: Right. So he ignored the comment about his sister. Good. Nick, did Jason complete Step 2b?

NICK: Uhm, let's see. Yeah, I guess he did because he told Mr. Adler that it pissed him off when he said that about his sister. So that's sort of saying how you feel.

TEACHER 1: Do you think he said it in a friendly way?

NICK: I don't know. Yeah, it probably was friendly. At least it was friendlier than screaming at him.

TEACHER 1: Okay, good. So far, we think Jason did a good job with each of these steps. How about Step 2c? Aaron, did Jason follow that step? . . .

The feedback activity moves quickly and ends with Jason evaluating his own performance in the role play. Role playing then continues with each student being provided an opportunity to role play the skill discussed that session. The session ends with the teacher handing out homework cards to be completed and signed by an adult prior to the next session. An example of one written on a 4" × 6" index card is provided in Figure 4.3. The purpose of assigning homework is to facilitate the use of this newly acquired skill in students' natural environments. The teacher is also in a position to periodically prompt and reinforce these behaviors as they occur in the classroom setting.

CONCLUSIONS

It is evident that most of the behavior of students with learning and behavior problems is under the influence of a complex array of events. In some instances, internal events such as

HOMEWORK CARD

Student _____ Date Assigned _____

Skill to be Practiced: <u>RESPONDING TO TEASING</u>

Date	Description of Incident	Student Response	Teacher Initials

FIGURE 4.3. Example of a homework card used in social skills training.

thoughts and emotions may be important antecedents to overt behaviors. Hence, it may be beneficial to target these areas and teach the child adaptive cognitive and emotional responses, as well as specific alternative coping skills for use in problem situations. The cognitive-based procedures discussed here are representative of the types of approaches that consider cognitions and emotions to be an important target for intervention. Cognitive-based self-management interventions have also been shown to be useful additions to contingency-based approaches in the treatment of a variety of academic and behavior problems in students.

5

Intervention Approaches for Students with Severe Disabilities

Self-management interventions have not been routinely applied to students with severe disabilities (Browder & Shapiro, 1985). There are at least three reasons for this situation. First, a general assumption exists that individuals with limited cognitive capacities will not be able to learn and use self-management procedures. Many assume that cognitive deficits result in reduced abilities to think and reason, and that these skills are necessary prerequisites for the development of self-management skills (Shapiro, 1981). However, research and clinical experience during the past decade suggests that individuals need not be excluded from implementing their own educational programming solely on the basis of their cognitive deficits. As stated by Browder and Shapiro (1985), "people do not need to reach a level of readiness to learn to manage their own behavior" (p. 206).

The second reason for the limited use of self-management with this population is that, historically, it was assumed that the presence of severe disabilities automatically meant the person would remain almost completely dependent on others throughout his or her life. Children with severe disabilities were often placed in institutions that provided them with little hope for acquiring the skills needed to live in a less restrictive setting. These individuals were not *expected* to achieve independence in most aspects of their daily lives. Hence, the teaching of skills of independence and self-reliance was not considered an appropriate goal. Today, we acknowledge that our reduced expectations for individuals with severe disabilities actually serves to increase their dependency. As we failed to provide them with opportunities to overcome their dependency, we actually perpetuated their problems rather than remediating them (Shapiro, 1981). Recently, the emphasis has been placed on preparing students with severe disabilities to be as independent as possible in various environments within their communities (Giangreco & Meyer, 1988). As self-management strategies are specifically designed to increase the skills of independence and self-reliance, they may be particularly useful with this population.

The final crucial reason for the limited application of self-management interventions to individuals with severe disabilities is that these interventions were initially designed to be used with individuals with mild, or no, disabilities. As described and demonstrated in the literature, they were not considered to be applicable to learners with severe disabilities. Self-instruction, which involves students making verbal statements to themselves, and self-monitoring activities that involve paper-and-pencil recording methods are examples of procedures considered to be inappropriate for use with this population. However, practitioners gradually began to examine the ways in which they could modify these and other procedures to allow students with more severe disabilities to participate in them. In addition, other aspects of self-management (e.g., preference assessment, choice making, picture cues) that were particularly relevant to the concerns of students with severe disabilities were emphasized.

We now have evidence that independence and self-management skills may be enhanced in students with severe disabilities through adapting self-management procedures. This is the case even though self-management interventions continue to be used primarily with those who have less severe disabilities. In fact, self-management interventions appear to be particularly appropriate and important for students with severe disabilities, given the values and goals surrounding the education of these students. For example, self-management interventions clearly hold promise as a means of increasing the opportunities for integrating these students into regular education settings. Since self-management strategies are generally designed to develop and teach independence skills, the routine use of these procedures in the classroom may help to reduce the amount of time teachers must spend individually with these children and thus increase the likelihood they will be successfully integrated into regular education settings (Shapiro, 1981).

Self-management interventions are also consistent with the set of values that have guided recent decisions about policy and practice in the field of severe disabilities. Among other things, this set of values emphasizes the worth of the individual regardless of his or her disabilities, the importance of focusing on abilities rather than disabilities, and the need to change schools so that they encourage the inclusion and participation of all children (Peck, 1991). As expressed by Guess and Siegel-Causey (1985), it is essential that persons with disabilities begin to be perceived by others as "self-directing and purposeful human beings, rather than mere objects of external manipulation" (p. 234). Self-management interventions that facilitate self-directing behavior and personal independence can play a useful role in promoting these values.

It is increasingly evident that self-management interventions are appropriate and important for students with severe disabilities. The purpose of this chapter is, first, to identify the characteristics of students with severe disabilities, since these must be considered when developing effective self-management interventions for these individuals. The most effective practices to date in the educational programming for these students are discussed in detail, as is the relevance of self-management interventions.

CHARACTERISTICS OF STUDENTS WITH SEVERE DISABILITIES

The term "severe disabilities" is broad and inclusive in that it is applied to those students with the most challenging educational needs, who have typically been excluded from the educational mainstream (Evans, 1991). According to the Education for All Handicapped Children Act (which was passed in 1975 and renamed the Individuals with Disabilities Education Act in 1990), students with severe disabilities are children and adolescents who, due to the extent of their problems, need special educational or other services to enhance the possibility for meaningful participation in society and self-fulfillment. These are individuals identified with such labels as autistic, severely retarded or severely intellectually disabled, multiply handicapped, or dually sensory impaired (Meyer, Peck, & Brown, 1991).

Most traditional definitions of severe disabilities have emphasized the negative characteristics and skill deficits of these individuals. In contrast, the definition adopted by the Association for Persons with Severe Handicaps in 1986 emphasizes the ability of these individuals to fully participate in community life with the proper support:

> The Association for Persons with Severe Handicaps addresses the interests of persons with severe handicaps who have traditionally been labelled as severely intellectually disabled. These people include individuals of all ages who require extensive ongoing support in more than one major life activity in order to participate in integrated community settings and to enjoy a quality of life that is available to citizens with fewer or no disabilities. Support may be required for life activities such as mobility, communication, self-care, and learning as necessary for independent living, employment, and self-sufficiency. (Meyer, Peck, & Brown, 1991, p. 19)

Although not emphasized in this statement, it is true that students with severe disabilities typically have fewer skills and appropriate social behaviors than their nondisabled peers

(Meyer et al., 1991). They also frequently present many of the most challenging behaviors (Horner, 1991).

Approximately 2% of the school-age population is identified as severely handicapped for the purposes of educational programming (Evans, 1991). Although these students are relatively few in number, they constitute a diverse population due to differences in the severity of their handicapping condition, their age, and their associated disabilities. Despite this diversity, there are a few characteristics that can be considered common among this student population. First, many of these students exhibit speech and language delays and deviations. They may have limited (or no) expressive language, limited language comprehension, poor articulation, and/or bizzare speech (e.g., echolalic speech, speech that is out of context, purposeless speech). As a result, these students may communicate through other behavioral, gestural, or vocal means (Mar, 1991). Hence, alternative forms of communication may need to be considered and incorporated into the self-management interventions designed for such students.

Second, many students with severe disabilities engage in aberrant, repetitive, or self-injurious behaviors (Koegel & Koegel, 1989). For example, it is not uncommon to see children with severe disabilities engaging in such behaviors as continuous rocking back and forth, repetitive flicking of their fingers in front of their eyes, or even hitting and biting themselves. Intense and prolonged temper tantrums may also occur (Evans, 1991). However, the presence of severe problem behaviors should not prevent attempts to implement self-management interventions. In fact, in some cases, one of the underlying functions of the problem behaviors may be controlling the behavior of others. If, through the implementation of self-management strategies, the student achieves a sense of control over his or her enviroment problem behaviors may actually be reduced.

Finally, since there is a relationship between the severity of the disability and the extent of physical problems, students with severe disabilities are likely to experience physical and health impairments. As many as 80% of individuals with severe disabilities have significant motor difficulties (i.e., poor or no ambulatory skills). Fine motor and perceptual–motor skills may also be limited (Hardman, Drew, Egan, & Wolf, 1990). Obviously, these types of physical disabilities require adaptations in programming. For example, in using self-monitoring with a student who has sensory or motor impairments, the self-monitoring device will need to be adapted so that the student is able to self-monitor easily (Browder & Shapiro, 1985). Although each of these characteristics require some type of adaptation, none precludes the use of self-management interventions entirely.

CHARACTERISTICS OF EDUCATIONAL PROGRAMS FOR STUDENTS WITH SEVERE DISABILITIES

Unlike students with mild or moderate disabilities, individuals with severe disabilities were routinely denied access to the public schools until the passage of P.L. 94-142 in 1975. These children were generally thought to be unable to benefit from educational programs, and it was assumed that most would remain dependent and institutionalized throughout their lives (Williams, Vogelsberg, & Schutz, 1985). More recently, philosophical, legal, and educational arguments have been made for integrated programming.

Educational practices viewed by the field as state-of-the-art (termed current best practices) emphasize the inclusion of students with severe disabilities in regular classrooms, as well as normalization of educational practices (i.e., use of educational practices and procedures typically used with regular education students). The ultimate aim of educational programs is to prepare students with severe disabilities for maximum participation in integrated community settings (Giangreco & Meyer, 1988). Although educators would like to see these students learn to be as independent as possible, it may not be possible for them to achieve absolute independence. Rather, the focus is on *partial participation* which emphasizes the value of some level of participation in activities as opposed to withholding it until mastery is achieved. Through partial participation in, and individualized adaptation to, activities in the severely disabled students' natural social environments, they may be able to acquire skills that will allow them to function in a wide range of settings that historically were closed to students with disabilities (Baumgart et al., 1982).

Self-management interventions provide an ideal means for encouraging students' partial participation in activities. Students may begin to participate at various stages of self-management programming as outlined by Litrownik, White, McInnis, and Licht (1984). According to these authors, the steps involved in teaching self-management include: (1) general assessment of multiple areas, (2) specification of desired outcome, (3) specification of the self-management process, (4) specific assessment of target behaviors, (5) training, and (6) evaluation. During an initial session, a student may, for example, participate in the selection of the specific responses to be self-managed through being exposed to choices and observed for preferences. Or, the teacher may ask the student for his or her preferences in the selection of specific self-management procedures to be used (Browder & Shapiro, 1985). No matter how students involve themselves initially, it probably will be necessary to shape the actual self-management skills over time. While a student initially may have to be taught to use picture prompts, eventually these could serve as a means for having the person schedule their own activities. Self-management interventions such as this one may actually provide educators with a means of putting the principle of partial participation into practice in the classroom. For a more in-depth discussion of the most highly effective practices in the education of students with severe disabilities, the interested reader is referred to such sources as Giangreco and Meyer (1988); Horner, Meyer, and Fredericks (1986); or Meyer (1985, 1987).

SELF-MANAGEMENT AND STUDENTS WITH SEVERE DISABILITIES

As described elsewhere in this book, self-management refers to the process of controlling one's own behavior through managing antecedent or consequent stimuli. Of the available strategies, the self-management of antecedent stimuli is especially useful with individuals with severe disabilities. These antecedent strategies can involve either self-generated or externally generated cues (Agran, Fodor-Davis, Moore, & Deer, 1989). For students with severe disabilities, *self-generated* cues such as brief self-instructions may be used, while *externally generated* cues such as picture prompts or choice-making strategies may be used. Consequent strategies such as self-monitoring have also been used successfully with individuals with severe disabilites. Although each of these strategies is discussed separately in this chapter, it should be noted that there is a recent interest in combining individual self-management procedures (Agran et al., 1989; Gifford, Rusch, Martin, & White, 1984; Wacker & Berg, 1986). This interest is based on the observation that, any one procedure may be inadequate to facilitate the development of generalized self-management skills for individuals with multiple disabilities. Instead, many advocate the use of packages comprised of a combination of self-management procedures, which are added as needed to maximize the effects for each individual student. The reader is encouraged to keep this in mind as individual self-management procedures are discussed later in this chapter.

As educators begin designing self-management strategies for individuals not traditionally included in self-management programs, several practical issues may arise (Browder & Shapiro, 1985):

1. *The initial step may involve actively teaching students to respond independently.* Some students with severe disabilities may engage in few, or no, independent adaptive responses. Many have long histories of waiting for a teacher to prompt every response. Others may engage in high rates of aberrant self-stimulatory behavior that interferes with independent adaptive responding. In such cases, an initial step in teaching the self-management of behavior may be simply to shape independent responding within a task or activity.

2. *The students' cognitive, physical, and sensory capabilities must be considered.* For example, with self-monitoring, the teacher must select or develop a self-recording device that can be used

by a student who may have minimal or no understanding of numerical concepts. Examples of such devices include rings on dowels, clickers, beaded bracelets, or marbles. When a student has a sensory or motor disability, the device will need to be adapted to incorporate a response the student makes or can easily learn to make.

3. *A decision must be made regarding the fading of self-management procedures.* Self-management strategies typically are viewed as a temporary means to achieve a desired objective (e.g., increased responding to tasks, reduction in aberrant behavior, increased work productivity). As the person begins to engage in the adaptive response independently, the self-management strategy may be faded. However, with students with severe disabilities, fading self-management procedures such as the use of a self-recording device may be neither necessary nor desirable since this could result in the loss of positive behavior gains. As an alternative, educators may wish to consider ways to make the procedure less intrusive over time to reduce the likelihood that it will interfere with community integration efforts.

4. *Self-management strategies must be adapted to those settings in which they are to be used.* As implied above, self-management procedures should be as unobtrusive as possible, especially when used in the community or in regular education settings. In a community recreational facility, a subtle recording device may assist a person in changing his or her behavior in an unobtrusive manner. In educational or home settings, the person may use picture prompts to learn a skill such as time management.

5. *Self-management strategies may be useful in programs designed to decelerate undesirable behavior.* Most practitioners focus on the use of self-management interventions to increase the independent occurrence of adaptive behaviors. However, there is some evidence to suggest that self-management strategies may also be effective in reducing a variety of aberrant behaviors (e.g., Gardner, Clees, & Cole, 1983; Gardner, Cole, Berry, & Nowinski, 1983; Morrow & Presswood, 1984). Thus, teachers should consider implementing self-management interventions to treat the excessive and inappropriate behavior of students with severe disabilities.

In summary, while some students may only be able to partially participate in their own behavior change programs, these individuals need not be excluded from the community or regular education settings regardless of their current skills or deficits. Specific self-management interventions such as self-instruction training, the use of picture prompts, choice making, and self-monitoring provide practitioners with valuable methods for encouraging student participation and independent functioning at various stages of instruction. Indeed, as Browder and Shapiro note, "Self-management training should be an extension of all instruction for community independence" (1985, p. 206).

SELF-INSTRUCTION TRAINING

Due to the nature of the strategy itself and its reliance on verbal stimuli, self-instruction training has typically involved children and adults of normal intelligence. However, when included as one aspect of a multicomponent intervention package, self-instruction training may also prove useful with individuals with severe disabilities. Aptly illustrating this, Keogh, Faw, Whitman, and Reid (1984) taught complex game playing skills to two adolescents with severe mental retardation. The training package consisted of teacher instructions, modeling, prompting, contingent praise, and self-verbalizations of game steps in a forward chaining procedure. Although the separate effects of the self-verbalizations were not evaluated, the boys did learn to self-instruct independently. The authors felt the self-statements were crucial to the success of the training package. Unfortunately, these skills failed to generalize to new games.

In a second example in which this strategy was included in a multicomponent package, self-instruction formed part of a social skills training package designed to increase the ability of five employees with moderate to severe intellectual disabilities to initiate conversations with their supervisors (Agran, Salzberg, & Stowitschek, 1987). Training resulted in the maintenance and generalization of the new skills. These examples would suggest that educators may wish to supplement traditional teaching procedures with a simple self-instruction component designed as a self-prompting strategy, with students who have verbal skills.

Self-instruction typically involves self-generated cues; that is, students are taught to verbalize statements that will cue appropriate responding. In an effort to adapt this procedure to students with severe disabilities, one group of investigators used prerecorded verbal prompts, an externally-generated cue, to facilitate student performance (Alberto, Sharpton, Briggs, & Stright, 1986). In this case, four high school students with severe mental retardation used a Walkman tape player that cued them to operate a washing machine, prepare a sandwich and cup of soup, or assemble a multipiece pipe unit. Instead of having the students generate the self-instructions, the tape provided the verbal prompts needed to complete the tasks at appropriately timed intervals. At specific points in the tape, the verbal prompts directed the students to stop the activity, survey his or her materials, and determine the accuracy of completed steps. The recorded prompts enabled the four students to acquire the new skills and, later, to perform these skills without the use of the tape player.

Although the procedure described above does not truly involve self-instruction, it provides an example of how the concept of self-instruction may be adapted for individuals with limited verbal skills. In this case, the tape recorder performed the function of instructing students to complete the various steps of the task. Obviously, the effect of this strategy was to facilitate the independent functioning of these students and thus move them closer to self-managing their own behavior. In this respect, it can be considered a useful strategy for promoting self-management in this population.

PICTURE PROMPTS

Another promising antecedent strategy that may enhance the self-management skills of students with severe disabilities is the use of picture prompts. Picture prompts are used to facilitate task performance by showing students a picture of each step of a task to be performed and then training them to use the pictures to independently guide their own performance on the task. Through teacher instructions, practice, and feedback, students are taught to imitate the performance depicted in a picture, turn to the next picture and imitate that performance, and so on, until the task is completed (Wacker & Berg, 1983).

It has been suggested that picture prompts establish a "look-then-do" sequence, which enables students to function more independently in their environments (Martin, Rusch, James, Decker, & Trtol, 1982). In addition, there are several other advantages to using picture prompts to modify the performance of students with severe disabilities have been suggested. These advantages include (1) cost effectiveness, since less time is needed to teach students to independently manage their own behavior, (2) the reduced need for teacher supervision, since students learn to use picture cues to guide their own behavior, and (3) the greater likelihood the behavior will be maintained and generalized since pictures provide stable cues that students can use to guide performance across time, settings, and tasks (Martin et al., 1982; Wacker & Berg, 1984).

In an early example of the use of picture prompts, picture recipe cards were used to successfully teach three adults with severe mental retardation to prepare simple foods (hot chocolate, Jell-O, and hot dogs) in a sheltered workshop setting (Robinson-Wilson, 1977). The visual cues consisted of hand-drawn picture recipe cards and color-coded stove dials. This suggests that even simple, low-budget picture prompts may serve to effectively guide student task performance.

Picture prompts have also been shown to aid in the completion of vocational tasks in educational settings. For example, Wacker and Berg (1983) used a sequence of black-and-white photographs to teach five high school students with moderate to severe mental retardation complex vocational tasks. A separate picture book was developed for each of the training tasks (a valve assembly and a circuit board assembly) and the generalization tasks (double valve assembly and a packaging task). The three-step training procedure involved:

1. Teaching students to turn the pages of the picture books.
2. Requiring them to correctly select the items pictured on each page.
3. Having them assemble the items shown in the photographs.

Results indicated that the picture cues also facilitated students' correct responding to the generalization tasks without additional training. This suggests that teaching students to use picture cues with one task may assist in the correct completion of other tasks using picture cues, even if the other tasks are unfamiliar to the student and have not been taught directly by the teacher.

These investigators also found that high school students with moderate to severe disabilities could use picture cues to set up work stations independently (Wacker & Berg, 1984). The task they were asked to do involved the correct placement of 18 valve assembly pieces or 20 packaging pieces across three work tables on an assembly line operation. Photographs were used to successfully guide students in the placement of the objects. Students were also able to successfully complete a new task with the use of picture cues appropriate for that task. Taken together, these two studies indicate that students with severe disabilities can be taught to function independently during each stage of a task, from setting up the work station to completing the task itself. Indeed, it is conceivable that students could use picture prompts to facilitate independent functioning during many, if not most, of the activities they are involved in throughout the day.

As an illustration of how picture prompts can be extended to other activities, Bambara and Ager (1992) used them to assist adults with moderate developmental disabilities in choosing and scheduling their desired leisure and recreational activities. Self-scheduling consisted of having each individual choose his or her desired leisure/recreational activities via picture cards and then place the cards in an activity book that provided space for each day of the week. Examples of the type of picture activity cards used in this study are provided in

Figure 5.1. Training for schedule implementation consisted of a daily prompt to look at the picture schedule plus a nightly review of the activities engaged in. All participants learned to independently self-schedule their leisure activities. In addition, the procedure resulted in substantial increases in the frequency and diversity of self-directed leisure activity, as well as increases in the novelty of activities. This suggests that, in addition to promoting task completion, picture prompts may also be a useful strategy for facilitating student involvement in appropriate leisure and recreational activities.

CHOICE MAKING

Within the growing body of literature that stresses the importance of increasing personal autonomy for individuals with severe disabilities, one area that has received a great deal of recent attention is choice making (Guess, Benson, & Siegel-Causey, 1985; Shevin & Klein, 1984; Zeph, 1984). The rationale and potential benefits of allowing individuals with severe disabilities to express preferences and make choices have been discussed from a number of different perspectives (Bannerman, Sheldon, Sherman, & Harchik, 1990; Guess et al., 1985; Shevin & Klein, 1984). First, implementing choice making is viewed as one way to enhance the quality of life of persons with severe handicaps (Parsons, Reid, Reynolds, & Bumgarner, 1990). For example, research indicates that an individual's overall satisfaction increases with expanded opportunities to pursue personal preferences (Musante, Gilbert, & Thibaut, 1983; Richter & Tjosvold, 1980). Thus, routinely providing individuals with severe disabilities opportunities to express their preferences by making selections from among several alternatives can be seen as one way to enhance their quality of life.

Second, it has been noted that individuals with severe disabilities are not provided with many choice-making opportunities (Dattilo & Rusch, 1985; Houghton, Bronicki, & Guess, 1987; Reid & Parsons, 1991). Given the importance of choice making and the relative lack of choice opportunities provided

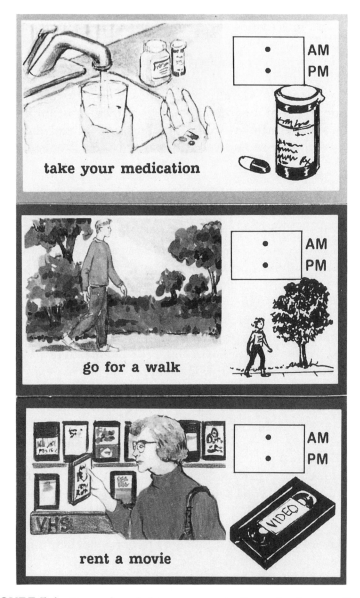

FIGURE 5.1. Examples of picture prompts. From Attainment Company, Inc., Verona, WI. Reprinted with permission.

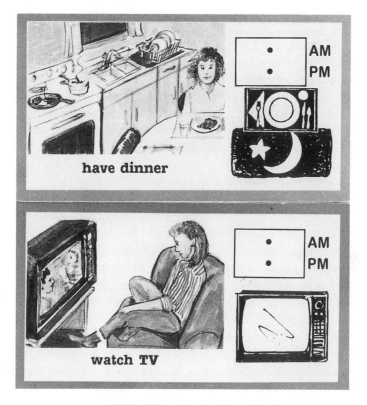

FIGURE 5.1. (*continued*)

to this population, researchers and practitioners have developed ways to increase choice for individuals with severe disabilities.

Overall, the effects of providing students with severe disabilities meaningful choice opportunities are positive. In addition to the benefits discussed above, it has been found that choice making helps to reduce social avoidance behavior (Koegel, Dyer, & Bell, 1987), increases spontaneous communication (Dyer, 1987; Peck, 1985), results in improved task performance (Mithaug & Mar, 1980; Parsons et al., 1990), and decreases serious problem behaviors (Dyer, Dunlap, & Winterling, 1990).

Methods for Assessing Choice and Preference

In many cases, personal preferences and choice-making skills must be assessed before meaningful choices can be offered to students with severe disabilities. Educational personnel involved with students with severe disabilities may encounter practical problems in attempting to assess preferences and choice-making skills in the classroom. A child with severe disabilities, who is suddenly provided with opportunities to choose from among several options, may fail to respond in a meaningful way (Mithaug & Hanawalt, 1978).

It is obvious that practitioners must find alternative methods for determining student preferences in cases such as this. In general, one of the most common assessment approaches with this population is to gather information through interviews with caregivers. Unfortunately, this approach may prove inaccurate as well. Research suggests that, compared with objective behavioral observations of children, information obtained through parental interviews may be inaccurate, even for children who present mild or no disabilities (Alessi, 1988). As this method of assessment is inaccurate for children with less severe problems, there is no reason to believe parental interview data would be any more accurate for students with severe disabilities. In fact, recent research has found that the subjective opinion of caregivers may not predict what students with severe disabilities will actually do when provided with a choice-making opportunity (Green, Reid, White, Halford, Brittain, & Gardner, 1988; Parsons & Reid, 1990). As the traditional approach of questioning caregivers does not appear to reliably predict what individuals with severe disabilities will actually choose, alternative methods must be sought.

As an alternative to traditional assessment approaches, Mithaug and colleagues (Mithaug & Hanawalt, 1978; Mithaug & Mar, 1980) developed a nonverbal method of assessing vocational preferences in persons with severe disabilities. Generally, this assessment procedure involved randomly pairing several tasks, and asking the student to select and work for several minutes on one task from each pair combination. Information gathered over several sessions was then used to determine individual client preferences. Although this method has been used primarily with adults (Green et al., 1988; Mithaug & Hanawalt, 1978; Mithaug & Mar, 1980; Parsons & Reid, 1990), it may also be appropriate for assessing preference and choice making in children within educational settings.

Mithaug and colleagues (Mithaug & Hanawalt, 1978; Mithaug & Mar, 1980) described the use of this nonverbal method to assess the task preferences of individuals with limited language skills and severe cognitive disabilities in a prevocational training classroom. The procedures involved the following steps:

1. Six tasks within the curriculum of the prevocational program were identified for use in the assessment. These included sorting, collating, stuffing, pulley assembly, flour-sifter assembly, and circuit board stuffing. Clients were familiar with each of the tasks prior to the assessment.

2. All possible pair combinations were identified for these tasks. The 6 tasks, presented 2 at a time, yielded a total of 15 pairs.

3. A tray containing a representative object from each of the two tasks was presented to the client. The placement of these objects on the tray (left or right) was random to control for the potential that a person would choose an item solely on the basis of its position.

4. The tray was placed on the table beside the client with the verbal prompt, "Pick one up, please."

5. After the client picked up one object from the tray, the tray was removed, the choice was recorded, and materials were supplied so that the client could perform the task for a 7-minute period.

6. At the end of the period, a buzzer sounded to indicate that no more work was to be done, and the clients left their work stations for a 2-minute break while data were recorded and the tray was prepared for the next choice.

7. The task selected during the trial just completed was paired at random with a different task. For example, if collating was chosen over stuffing on Trial 1, collat-

ing was paired at random with one of the remaining four tasks on Trial 2. If collating was chosen again over another task, it was paired at random with one of the remaining three tasks on the next trial. As long as the person continued to select collating, this procedure was repeated for all possible pairs. On the sixth trial, a new pair combination was selected at random and the procedures repeated.

8. The choices clients made regarding the task objects were scored when they picked up one of the objects from the tray and set it on the table. A choice was not recorded when a client picked up an object and then put it back on the tray.

9. Assessment information consisted of determining the percentage of times a client chose a particular task when it was paired with every other task.

10. All 15 possible pair combinations were presented randomly every 2 days for a period of 34 days, with clients making 8 selections on the first day and the remaining seven selections on the second day.

It is important to note that the assessment procedure required that individuals learn the relationship between picking up a task object from the tray and working on the task represented by that object. Depending upon a variety of factors, including the person's level of functioning and familiarity with the tasks, multiple experiences might be required before he or she associated the choice objects with the corresponding tasks. Hence, education practitioners should keep this in mind when conducting a preference assessment and extend the assessment activities as long as needed to ensure that students actually understand the choice–consequence relationship. In addition, initial preference information may be less useful for certain individuals than information obtained later in the assessment process when they begin to understand the choice–consequence relationship.

This type of nonverbal assessment can be adapted for classroom use to assess student preferences for objects or activities within that environment. The most obvious application of this method is in the area of assessing student preference for various functional academic or vocational tasks. In addition, this assessment method has been used to determine children's preferences for various food and beverage items (Parsons & Reid, 1990; Sigafoos & Dempsey, 1992), as well as other potential reinforcers (Green et al., 1988). For example, Sigafoos and Dempsey (1992) had teachers provide children with multiple disabilities opportunities for choice making in their classroom. The assessment procedure involved the following steps:

1. The children were assessed as a group during the morning snack time. These assessment sessions occurred two or three times per week.
2. During each trial, the teacher placed a small portion of a food item (e.g., cake, cookie) and a beverage item (e.g., milk, juice) on the child's wheelchair lap tray or, if the child did not use a wheelchair, in the teacher's hands. The left/right placement of items was altered randomly across opportunities.
3. The teacher called the child's attention to the items and instructed him or her to make a choice (e.g., "Look, Ruth, here is some cake [pointing to the cake] and some juice [pointing to the cup of juice]. What would you like?").
4. Any indication during the next 15 seconds that a choice was made followed by giving the child that item, and observing and recording his or her acceptance or refusal of it. Items refused were withdrawn immediately.
5. This procedure was repeated with each child until all children had experienced five choice opportunities during that particular session.

An important consideration in assessing students with severe disabilities for their preferences is that individual students may have idiosyncratic ways of indicating choice. For example, rather than reaching for an item, some students may indicate a preference by motioning toward one of the two offered items, looking at one of the items for several seconds, or smiling or vocalizing while looking at one of the items. Ambiguities are certain to arise in preference assessment since these individuals may not exhibit precise verbal responses, facial expressions, task avoidance behaviors, and other means by which preferences are typically communicated (Mithaug & Hanawalt, 1978; Shevin & Klein, 1984). As with other types of assessment of this population, familiarity with the student may be an important factor in obtaining a reliable preference assessment.

Providing Choices in the Classroom

Although providing choices to students with severe disabilities may appear to be a relative simple activity, in fact, choice is often not provided in the classroom. Students typically have little or no input in decisions regarding their educational goals or the procedures that are used to teach them (Bannerman et al., 1990; Guess et al., 1985; Shevin & Klein, 1984). Educators may teach behaviors with little or no regard for students' preferences or past learning in a particular academic area. Indeed, choice making skills are usually not actively taught.

The absence of choice making in educational programs for students with severe disabilities cannot be blamed solely on the teachers who instruct these students. Teacher training programs historically have emphasized the importance of establishing control over student behavior, and not the importance of providing students with choices. As a result of this focus, teachers may have thought little about the concept of choice or about how to incorporate it in the curriculum. In fact, there does not appear to be an accepted definition of "choice" or "choice making" in the literature. Brigham (1979) defined choice as "the opportunity to make an uncoerced selection from two or more alternative events, consequences, or responses" (p. 132). However, the word "uncoerced" implies freedom from external influence and behavior analysts may argue that choice is never free (Bannerman et al., 1990). Perhaps the following is a more descriptive definition of choice: "The act of an individual's selection of a preferred alternative from among several familiar options" (Shevin & Klein, 1984, p. 160). To meet this definition, (1) the person must be able to reliably express personal preferences, and (2) the options must be familiar to the person. The latter requires that the person have experience with the various options on several occasions prior to offering him or her a choice between them.

There are several compelling arguments in favor of fostering a choice-making curriculum for students with severe disabilities. Research studies with a number of different populations have indicated positive effects result from choice making (Bannerman et al., 1990). For example, in studies that investigated whether individuals prefer choice situations to nonchoice situations, individuals frequently selected the former. One study found that adolescents with developmental disabilities who engaged in stereotypic rocking more frequently chose a chair in which they could rock themselves than a chair rocked by an adult at the same rate. The only difference between the two conditions was whether or not the adolescent controlled the rocking (Buyer, Berkson, Winnega, & Morton, 1987).

A second finding was that individuals tended to participate more in activities if choice opportunities were available. For example, adolescent and young adult males with mild to moderate mental retardation who were given an opportunity to choose the T-shirts they wanted to iron increased their participation in the subsequent ironing activity (Rice & Nelson, 1988). A related finding was that opportunities to make choices improve task performance. As an example, children's performance on an art task improved when they were allowed to choose their own art materials (Amabile & Gitomer, 1984).

Finally, providing choice opportunities may also serve to reduce problem behaviors. For example, in one study, children with autism exhibited fewer problem behaviors (e.g., aggression, self-injury) when they could choose tasks, materials, and reinforcers than when an adult made these choices (Dyer, Dunlap, & Winterling, 1989). In another example of this, children with autism demonstrated less social avoidance (e.g., looking and moving away) when they were engaged in activities they preferred (Koegel et al., 1987). In summary, the research indicates that individuals generally prefer situations in which they are provided with a choice. Further, choice making may serve to increase participation and reduce problem behaviors.

The above research suggests that the potential benefits of

providing students with severe disabilities choices in the classroom far outweigh any extra time and effort that may be required to help them learn to make choices. This does not imply, however, that educators should sit back and allow students total freedom to design their own programming. On the contrary, educational teams should find ways to integrate choice making into the established curriculum. Bannerman et al. (1990) suggested the following ways to accomplish this goal for students with severe disabilities:

1. *Educators should emphasize teaching student-preferred functional behaviors.* A number of functional behaviors can be identified for possible focus within the curriculum. Rather than relying solely on educators' judgments in selecting the specific functional behaviors or skills to be taught, student preference could be considered as well. If high preference behaviors are targeted, eventually students will be equipped with a repertoire of appropriate, as well as preferred, behaviors from which to make choices.

2. *Students should have input in decisions about how skills will be taught.* Interdisciplinary teams should make decisions about a student's future only after considering student preferences. The nonverbal preference assessment procedure described in the previous section may be useful in accomplishing this goal.

3. *Students should be taught how to choose.* Examples of curricula available for teaching students with severe disabilities choice making include: (1) a leisure skills training program that includes suggestions for teaching choice making (Wuerch & Voeltz, 1982); (2) a program for teaching youth with autism to choose leisure materials (Henning & Dalrymple, 1986); and (3) an instructional curriculum for teaching choice making in everyday situations (Guess & Helmstetter, 1986). Additional suggestions about how to prepare students for making choices include: (4) teaching concepts like "choose," "now," "later," "I want," and "I do not want" (Shevin & Klein, 1984); (5) teaching the functional use of "yes" and "no" (Guess, Sailor, & Baer, 1976); and (6) teaching more complex decision making by listing options, discussing advantages and disadvantages of each option, and indicating which option might be the best (Reese, 1986).

4. *Students at every level of functioning should be provided with opportunities to make choices during and between scheduled activities.* Each student's daily schedule of activities should be set up to allow time for making choices of various kinds (e.g., choosing activities between tasks, choosing the order in which activities will be completed, choosing the location of activities). This is especially important for students who are still learning about the choice–consequence relationship.

As indicated by these suggestions, integrating choice in the daily curriculum requires both systematic teaching of new skills, and the provision of opportunities to practice these skills in and outside the classroom. Students can learn to make choices only by making their own decisions and experiencing the consequences of these decisions (Kamii, 1991). However, providing students with severe disabilities with meaningful choice opportunities throughout the day may be a difficult task for the teacher. In the early stages, it may require considerable creativity and effort. Shevin and Klein (1984) suggest several types of choices that may be useful in educational settings. An important aspect to consider is that the teacher must be prepared to accept the option the student selects, for each choice presented. The various types of choices include:

1. *Choice among various objects or activities.* The teacher might ask the student, for example, "Would you like to use the red marker or the blue marker?"
2. *Choice of whether or not to engage in an activity.* The teacher might ask the student, for example, "Do you want to count money?" An answer of "No" by the student should then be accepted by the teacher.
3. *Choice of when to terminate an activity.* The teacher might ask, for example, "Do you want to do that again?" An answer of "No" should then be accepted. In other cases, students may indicate during an activity that they wish to do something else or that they wish to continue an activity the teacher wants to terminate.
4. *Choice of partners for activities.* The teacher might ask, for example, "Who would you like to work with?"

In addition to these, choices may be integrated in a variety of other areas. Examples of additional areas that might be included are (1) the sequencing of steps within a task (e.g., "Which step do you want to do first?"); (2) the scheduling of daily activities (e.g., "Which activity do you want to do next?"); (3) the timing of the onset of a scheduled activity (e.g., "Do you want to start now or in 5 minutes?"); (4) where the activity is performed (e.g., "Do you want to work here or at the table over there?"); (5) the task materials that are used in performing the activity (e.g., "Do you want to use the drawing or photographs?"); (6) the amount of assistance provided (e.g., "Do you need help or would you like to try to do this by yourself?"), and (7) the working conditions (e.g., "Do you want to work alone or with the group?").

The options for providing choice are virtually unlimited. Almost any teacher statement can be restated in such a way as to include a choice option. Even with activities in which choice making does not seem to apply (e.g., putting on a coat to go outside in cold weather), simple choices may be found (e.g., "Do you want to get your coat or should I?", "Do you want to start with this arm or that arm?", "Do you want to wear your collar up or down?", "Do you want to zip the rest of the way or not?"). These are merely provided as examples of choices that could be generated surrounding a relatively simple, routine activity. Obviously, it would not be advisable to inundate a student with *all* of these choices on any one occasion! Providing one or two choices during an activity of this nature, and varying the types of choices provided across days, is a more advisable approach.

The teacher must also consider the age and ability level of the student in relation to the significance and/or risk of the choice when implementing choice making for the classroom (Shevin & Klein, 1984). Not all choices are appropriate for all students. For example, it may be appropriate to provide a choice of snack items to a young child, but not a choice between wearing a lightweight jacket or a snowsuit when the temperature outside is below freezing. In fact, because of the risks associated with wearing a lightweight jacket in freezing weather, the latter may never be an appropriate choice. As students increase in age and ability level, they may also benefit from expanded choice options across a number of domains. Older students, for example, should be given opportunities to express personal preferences for vocational activities and to select vocational sites that they would like to work in. The key is to present students with options within the parameters of acceptable behavior.

SELF-MONITORING

Although each of the self-management strategies described to this point involve intervention *prior to* the occurrence of a target behavior, the consequent strategy of self-monitoring may also be useful in educational programming for students with severe disabilities. Unfortunately, we have few examples of the application of self-monitoring to individuals with severe disabilities, as a majority of the self-monitoring studies have focused on individuals with mild, or no, disabilities (Browder & Shapiro, 1985). Hence, relatively little is known about the ability of students with severe disabilities to self-monitor or the effects of self-monitoring on their behavior. In addition, studies that target individuals with severe disabilities have typically involved adults in sheltered workshop settings, although similar techniques may be appropriate for use in educational settings. For example, Hanel and Martin (1980) used self-monitoring (with self-reinforcement) to increase the production rates of eight workshop clients with mild to severe mental retardation. A marble-dispensing device was used to help these clients self-monitor each task completed; they exchanged marbles for money at the end of each session. Productivity increased 43% over baseline levels using this strategy. It is easy to see how a similar strategy could be applied to vocational or prevocational tasks in an educational setting. The advantage of this type of self-monitoring procedure for this population is that it involves a very concrete, and potentially reinforcing, mechanism for self-monitoring. For some students, this type of strategy may be preferable to the more abstract pencil-and-paper methods that have been shown to be so effective with students with less severe disabilities (see Chapter 3).

While the target behavior in this example was task completion, the more common educational strategy of having students self-monitor on-task or attending behavior has also been used successfully with this population. For example, Rudrud, Rice, Robertson, and Olson (1984) in a work activity center taught 16 clients who had mild to severe disabilities to self-record on-task behavior when they heard a prerecorded tone. Following this procedure, work production increased 11.2%. In a slightly different example in which the target behavior was job initiative, individuals with severe disabilities were taught to mark a recording pad whenever they noticed a job initiative situation and each time they responsed to it. Participants were also praised for self-monitoring and given tokens that were exchangeable for money. This procedure, combined with discrimination training and role playing, increased the job initiative skills in these sheltered workers.

Although self-monitoring has produced positive behavior change when used with individuals with severe disabilities, there is evidence that, in some cases, the addition of reinforcement procedures may be necessary to achieve and maintain desired levels of performance. For example, Mace, Shapiro, West, Campbell, and Altman (1986) investigated the role of self-monitoring and reinforcement with three sheltered workshop employees with moderate to severe disabilities. Prior to the study, each person was taught how to self-monitor. Following baseline, two workers were given contingent praise and money for reaching individualized production rates that were above their usual rates. Next, these two participants were introduced to self-monitoring. This increased their production rate further and decreased its variability across days. When reinforcement was withdrawn, performance rates returned to baseline levels. Reinstatement of reinforcement once again increased their performance rates. The intervention order was different for the third worker but the results were similar. The addition of reinforcement once again increased productivity over that observed with self-monitoring alone. For these individuals, adding reinforcement to the self-monitoring procedure was needed to achieve increased production. Self-monitoring alone was not sufficient to have the desired effects on work productivity. This would suggest that educators should include a reinforcement contingency with self-monitoring interventions for students with severe disabilities to increase the likelihood these strategies will result in positive effects.

CONCLUSION

The empirical literature devoted to the use of self-management strategies with students with severe disabilities is limited. This limitation is evident both in the small number of studies available, and in the restrictions in types of settings and ages of participants found within them. Indeed, few investigations have involved children with severe disabilities in educational settings. Further, while the literature suggests positive effects result from the use of these strategies, independent contributions of specific self-management components are often lacking. In many cases, self-managment procedures are embedded with other procedures in a multicomponent intervention package, and thus their effects cannot be determined.

Despite these limitations, the results of these initial studies are encouraging. Many individuals with severe disabilities can learn to self-monitor their behavior and, as a result, increase their task performance. Students are also able to learn to make choices and express their preferences, the benefits of which may be tremendous. Even self-instruction strategies may be modified for use with individuals with severe disabilities. The interventions described here are only representative of the types of self-management strategies that may be used successfully with this population. Creative educators are certain to discover countless new ways to apply and adapt the concepts of self-management to students with severe disabilities. The shift from external teacher management toward self-management illustrated by these strategies represents a major departure from the practices of the past.

6

Implementation Issues

As described in previous chapters, self-management interventions generally involve teaching children to use strategies that will increase their appropriate academic or social behaviors and/or decrease their inappropriate classroom behaviors. It is also useful to view self-management skills as on a continuum. In other words, it is evident that the locus of control of behavior is a matter of degree. As children move along this continuum from external teacher control toward self-management, they assume more and more responsibility for completing various activities. But seldom is any behavior under total external or total internal influence, for no one is ever "self-managed" in an absolute sense. Thus, a reasonable initial objective may be to introduce self-management components one at a time into the classroom routine or to introduce self-management strategies to only a few students at a time. As these activities are assimilated into the daily routine, self-management can be extended to other areas or other students. Self-management should not be viewed in all-or-nothing terms, but rather should be incorporated by gradually transferring responsibilities and offering more choices to students.

The process of shifting from an external teacher-management system to a self-management paradigm may be difficult to accomplish in some cases. A number of obstacles may be encountered such as teacher or student resistance. Also, to maximize the likelihood of successful outcomes, it is important to address issues such as how best to assess student behavior, the process of determining what type of self-management intervention will most benefit a particular student, and training for generalization of behavior change. The purpose of this chapter is to provide practitioners with practical suggestions for developing and implementing self-management interventions in school settings.

DEALING WITH TEACHER RESISTANCE

The traditional model of service delivery in the classroom is one of teacher management. This model places the teacher in charge of all major curriculum and classroom-management decisions. From this perspective, one measure of teacher success is how well students learn to sit quietly, comply with teacher directions and requests, raise hands to speak, and generally obey other classroom rules. Student input is sought infrequently and students are generally allowed little control. Thus, the teacher-management model assigns an authoritarian role to the teacher and a relatively passive, accepting role to the students.

Many teachers who were trained in this model are comfortable with it and feel no need to change. Others, however, believe there are benefits to be gained from more active student participation and involvement in decision making. These teachers may already be implementing some of the intervention strategies suggested in this book. In either case, it is important to recognize that instructors' attitudes toward the traditional teacher-management model will determine to some extent how receptive they are to self-management interventions. Unlike with many other interventions, the teacher must come to view students as participants in their own educational environment rather than as passive recipients of knowledge. The role of the teacher becomes one of offering learning experiences in which students assume increasing responsibility for their own behavior and for planning their future (Kanfer & Gaelick, 1986).

Another reason teacher attitudes are important is the increasing recognition in the behavioral literature that teacher attitudes toward classroom interventions determine to a large extent whether the interventions will ultimately be successful (e.g., Martens et al., 1985; Witt, 1986; Witt et al., 1984). This factor may be especially critical for self-management interventions, since a decrease in the level of teacher control is of central importance. In conclusion, if self-management interventions are to succeed, the teacher must be open to the idea of having students assume some of the responsibilities previously reserved for the teacher.

If this type of open attitude is not in place, it may be useful to attempt to cultivate it. Engaging a teacher in discussions about the importance of actively teaching students to assume responsibility and providing educational experiences designed to foster independence may be all that is needed. Another approach may be to suggest implementing a simple self-management strategy (e.g., self-monitoring) that is likely to produce positive results, and to use its success as an example of the benefits of self-management (e.g., requires less teacher time, enhances student motivation). Self-management interventions could also be promoted by other teachers who have used them and have experienced their benefits. These teachers may be asked to talk with others and perhaps share their results informally or at a formal meeting.

It is important to recognize that, despite such efforts, there will be teachers who will remain resistant to the concept of self-management. Although there is little question that fostering self-management skills in students is the goal for most every teacher, there may be a difference of opinion in how to go about teaching students to become more self-reliant. In light of the research which suggests that teacher attitudes greatly influence the effectiveness of interventions, forcing the issue by having a resistant teacher implement a self-management strategy is probably not productive. It may be more beneficial with this type of teacher to simply focus on an intervention that has a greater likelihood of being implemented consistently and, perhaps, revisit the concept of self-management at some time in the future.

ASSESSING STUDENT PROBLEMS

The careful assessment of student problems is obviously a critical factor in the ultimate success of a program. As with any behavioral intervention, a thorough understanding of the problem behavior should precede and dictate the selection of a treatment strategy, so that it will be the most appropriate for remediating that behavior. In fact, the primary objective of behavioral assessment is to obtain information from which a child-specific intervention program can be devised. For example, a diagnostic behavioral assessment may determine that a child's aggression toward others is an emotional, impulsive response which is triggered by specific peer actions. In this case, a stress-inoculation program designed to treat both the child's cognitive and affective responses to the action and to teach specific coping responses may be more appropriate than, for example, a simple self-monitoring or self-reinforcement procedure. Thus, a critical first step is to gather information concerning the factors that underlie, strengthen, and maintain a student's academic or behavior problem.

More specifically, the process of assessment typically involves the activities of (1) gathering information about variables that potentially augment the problem, and (2) developing hypotheses about specific contributing factors using this information. The information-gathering stage may include assessment of variables involved in the instigation of problem behaviors (e.g., external environmental events, personal characteristics), as well as factors contributing to the acquisition and persistent recurrence of these problem behaviors (e.g., positive reinforcement, negative reinforcement). Assessment information may be obtained through direct observation of the child in the classroom, review of case records, exposure to analog situations, and/or interviews with him or her, teachers, family members, or peers.

A variety of hypotheses about factors contributing to a

problem behavior may lead to the selection of a self-management intervention. For example, when a student's disruptive
behavior is thought to be maintained by contingent positive
consequences (e.g., teacher feedback, peer attention), the intervention may include approaches designed to teach and
strengthen skills that would serve as alternatives to the disruptive behavior. The child may be taught social skills that can be
used to produce the same or similar reinforcing consequences.
With another child, disruptive behavior may be functional in
reducing or terminating difficult task demands. In this case,
disruptive behavior may represent a form of escape-motivated
behavior, which is maintained by negative reinforcement (e.g.,
Carr & Newsom, 1985; Carr, Newsom, & Binkhoff, 1980). This
hypothesis supports the inclusion of intervention approaches
such as (1) removing or reducing the aversiveness of task demands, and (2) teaching the child specific problem-solving, or
other self-management, skills that can be used to eliminate or
minimize the effects of the aversive conditions. In a third example, disruptive behavior that occurs following peer teasing
may be thought to reflect a skill deficit. In other words, the
child just does not know what else to do when he or she is pro-
voked. This may lead to the design and implementation of a
skills training program that may include both contingency-
based and cognitive-based approaches.

In each of these cases, the hunches about the factors maintaining problem behaviors may lead to the development of
self-management interventions that are designed to teach new
skills and behaviors. Even in instances in which it is difficult to
establish the specific factors that serve to instigate or strength-
en and maintain a student's problem behavior, a variety of skill
development procedures can potentially effect the problem
behavior. A number of recent studies have demonstrated the
reduction of serious problem behaviors through the developing and/or strengthening of alternative social, coping, and other self-management skills (e.g., Bird, Dores, Moniz, & Robinson, 1989; Carr & Durand, 1985; Carr et al., 1980). In each
of these studies, a skill deficit rationale guided the selection of
the intervention procedures.

SELECTING SPECIFIC
INTERVENTION STRATEGIES

As previously described, the ultimate objective of assessment activities is to provide sufficient information for developing child-specific intervention procedures consistent with the hypotheses generated. Especially important in this assessment process is the gathering of information on the presence or absence of specific social, coping, and other self-management skills, as well as on the child's cognitive skills and abilities. This type of information will be the most useful in determining what type of self-management intervention will most benefit a particular student.

Although some self-management strategies can be employed with virtually all students, other approaches are useful only with students who possess particular characteristics. For example, self-monitoring procedures have been employed successfully with a wide range of populations of children and adolescents (Gardner & Cole, 1988; Shapiro & Cole, 1992). Although there are important issues to consider when children are self-monitoring, such as making clear which behavior is being targeted for monitoring and targeting only age-appropriate behaviors, children of all ages, ability level and handicapping conditions have used this procedure successfully.

On the other hand, most cognitive-based procedures (e.g., self-instruction, stress-inoculation, problem-solving), by their very nature, require that students already possess certain skills. As these strategies rely heavily on verbal and cognitive reasoning skills, they obviously have limited usefulness for very young children or students with severe cognitive disabilities. However, they may be very appropriate for use with regular education children and adolescents who are experiencing problems.

In addition to these general guidelines, practitioners may find that individual students react very differently to self-management procedures. Some students who have questionable prerequisite skills may, when provided with training in a self-management strategy, do much better than predicted. These students may find "being in control" to be such a reinforcing activity that they become highly motivated to participate and, as a result, perform better academically. For other children, self-management activities may actually prove to be a distraction, which interferes with their academic performance. Thus, although assessment information is helpful in the process of matching an intervention to a child, supplementing this information with pilot trials of specific procedures is recommended.

FACILITATING STUDENT COOPERATION

As previously discussed, teacher cooperation is essential for the success of self-management interventions. It is equally important, however, for students to be motivated to participate in the self-management activities. The emphasis on student responsibility in intervention requires that the child have, or develop, a strong desire to take on more responsibility and ultimately to change his or her behavior. Therefore, a critical task of the instructor is to motivate the student to actively participate in the behavior change process. In contrast with traditional teacher-managed programs based solely on environmental control, the early phase of self-management interventions is designed to help the student accept the need for change and to develop clear objectives for intervention (Kanfer & Gaelick, 1986). It is important to note, however, that without established incentives for change and environments that will continue to support and reinforce changes that do occur, behavior change cannot be expected to be maintained over time.

An important consideration in facilitating student cooperation, and one that is often overlooked in the self-management literature, is the student's *perception* of control. If a child continues to perceive him- or herself as being controlled by the instructor (e.g., teacher, school psychologist, counselor), even though he or she is being given responsibility for some of the program's activities, the active cooperation necessary to teach self-management and accomplish the intervention goals may fail to occur (Kanfer & Gaelick, 1986). Instead, the intervention effort may result in the child's resistance and lack of co-operation. Many of the self-management strategies described in previous chapters are based on the assumption that the instructor will play only a temporary and supportive role in guiding the child toward changing his or her behavior. Although it may be difficult for many who are used to "being in charge" or "maintaining control" in classrooms to assume a less powerful role, it is essential for program success. Instructors must, from the beginning, view themselves merely as facilitators or motivators, and seek to gain student input in all critical aspects of the program. This is especially true for older children and adolescents who may be generally resistant to adult intervention. Students of all ages and ability levels are much more likely to be successful if they have a perception of "ownership" of the self-management program.

To further enhance student cooperation, it is important that the self-management procedure is age-appropriate and motivating to the individual student. For example, in self-monitoring interventions, typically a prerecorded tone or beep is used to cue students to monitor and record their behavior. While this may work with many students, the motivation of younger students may be enhanced by substituting silly noises for the tones. Older students, on the other hand, may prefer musical interludes of 5–10 seconds of contemporary music as an alternative to the tones. The process of designing interventions should be flexible enough to meet the needs of individual students.

TRAINING STUDENTS TO USE SELF-MANAGEMENT

In addition to enhancing motivation, another primary role of the instructor is to help the student acquire those skills needed to implement the self-management strategies, and as a consequence produce change in the target behavior. The available research on simple self-management procedures such as self-monitoring suggest that training improves self-monitoring accuracy, especially in students with various handicapping conditions (e.g., Robertson et al., 1979; Shapiro et al., 1981). With more complex and comprehensive cognitive-based procedures such as social problem-solving and stress-inoculation training, rehearsal is an essential and integral part of the intervention. For all self-management interventions, sufficient time should be devoted to training in the procedure to ensure that students understand and are able to incorporate the strategies in their daily routine.

In addition to the initial training sessions, periodic booster sessions should be provided to ensure that students are using the self-management strategy properly and to avoid their straying from the original intent of the procedure. These booster sessions may also serve to enhance student morale and motivation to participate. Finally, booster sessions may serve to remind instructors of the objectives of the program and to focus on the specific strategies the students were supposed to have acquired.

TRAINING FOR GENERALIZATION

It is clear that an intervention that focuses only on the learning and performance of a specific behavior in a particular setting is inadequate. The transfer of skills to new settings and new situations, the generalization of skills to new behaviors, and the durability of behavior change across time are just as important. It is critical to consider these issues when designing a self-management intervention so that training can be structured to foster maintenance and generalization.

A primary factor in facilitating generalization is the training situation itself. Ideally, training should take place in the actual physical setting in which the behavior is likely to occur. In many cases, this means it would be preferable to conduct the training in the child's classroom, rather than in another location in the school. If this is not possible, the more similar the training setting to the natural setting in which the behaviors usually occur, the greater the odds that the students will perform the learned behaviors in that setting.

Second, when teaching self-management skills to children, it is useful to state directly the importance of applying what they have learned in the training setting to new situations with new and different problems. Although it is tempting to assume the child understands this and will do this automatically, many times generalization must be actively prompted, especially with young children or children with disabilities. In the area of self-instruction, for example, it is known that these skills may not occur automatically outside the training setting. Thus, instructors may need to actively teach self-instruction in each targeted academic subject area. Prompting the child with questions such as, "Where else could you do this?", "How will you handle this next time?", or "Did you use self-instructions in math class today?" may also help to facilitate the transfer of self-management behaviors to other situations or settings.

In addition, because repeated practice is important when facilitating the transfer of newly acquired skills, it is useful to enlist the help of other individuals from the child's environment (e.g., parents, peers, etc.). Even though behaviors may be correctly performed in a training situation, they probably will not be strong enough to replace the old, well-established responses if they have not been practiced and reinforced frequently outside the situation. For these reasons, although familial cooperation and involvement in the program is not always feasible, it is highly desirable whenever possible. For example, it may be useful to organize a parent group designed to focus on those features of the training program their children are receiving so that parents can prompt and reinforce the new behaviors (Kendall & Braswell, 1985). In another example, parents may be encouraged to praise their child for engaging in self-instructional behavior while completing his or her homework.

An additional powerful source of influence is a student's peers. Strategies such as peer monitoring of self-monitored behavior or peer tutoring of academic subjects often helps to facilitate the maintenance and generalization of self-managed behaviors. An example of a more elaborate program that combines self-management and peer interventions is Reciprocal Peer Tutoring (RPT; Fantuzzo & Rohrbeck, 1992). RPT combines opportunities for students to make choices and student management, with interdependent group-reward contingencies and reciprocal peer teaching. This type of program capitalizes on the advantages of self-management and peer-mediated interventions and can be implemented on a classwide basis.

RESERVATIONS AND COMMON PITFALLS

The self-management model provides a useful alternative to the teacher-management approach to classroom interventions. However, it is apparent that its application to the academic and behavior problems of *all* children would prove unworkable and, for some children, might even be detrimental. Self-management interventions are not appropriate for every child, and some specific strategies meet the needs of individual students better than others. A common mistake is to view self-management strategies as static, inflexible procedures that must be adhered to by students if the procedures are to be successful. A more productive approach is to view these strategies as a framework from which to design individualized interventions for particular students or groups of students. Procedures should be designed to fit the environment, rather than changing the environment to fit a rigid set of procedures.

Just as with external management approaches, self-management interventions typically fail due to a lack of environmental support, a lack of adequate training in the intervention procedures, or a lack of sufficient incentives and reinforcement for attempting to change (Kanfer & Gaelick, 1986). Suggestions for avoiding each of these pitfalls have been provided in this chapter. It is important to note the similarities between external management and self-management interventions in their reliance on external factors for long-term behavior change. It is incorrect to assume that, because students are learning skills for managing certain aspects of their behavior, external reinforcement for behavior is no longer necessary. Self-management strategies are seen as a complement to, not a replacement for, external reinforcement procedures already in place in the child's natural environment.

7

Case Illustrations

As is evident from material presented throughout this book, self-management procedures have been applied to a large number of school-based problems. This includes difficulties in both academic and nonacademic areas. In this chapter, a series of cases will be presented to further illustrate these procedures. Each of these cases represent the actual implementation of self-management stategies with children within school-based settings.

ACADEMIC SKILLS PROBLEMS

Case 1: David—Self-Managing Spelling Performance

Background

David was a fifth-grade student classified as having Serious Emotional Disturbance (SED). He was currently being instructed completely within the mainstream environment, with the addition of consultative support from a special education teacher. He was referred to the school psychologist because, in addition to his ongoing behavior problems, David was experiencing academic difficulties in the areas of spelling and reading.

While in the third grade, David was initially placed in a self-contained classroom for children with SED due to his teachers' ongoing reports of aggression, anxiety, and poor self-image. He was diagnosed as having Attention-deficit Hyperactivity Disorder (ADHD) at that time. Over the past year, David had made excellent progress, resulting in his being mainstreamed for all subjects. However, his teachers had recently reported that he was again having great difficulty completing his work due to high levels of distractibility.

Initial Assessment

An initial assessment of David's spelling skills was conducted prior to beginning the intervention program. At that time, David was being instructed at the second-grade level of the spelling series. Results of the assessment suggested that this was an accurate placement for David at that time. Shortly after the assessment, David completed this book and was moved to the second-grade level book of a more challenging spelling series. An assessment of his spelling performance using this series was again conducted. Results showed that David's performance was instructional at both the second- and third-grade levels of the series. As a result, it was recommended to his teacher that David be instructed in the third-grade level of the new curriculum.

Instructional Arrangements

Spelling instruction in David's classroom was primarily provided through independent seatwork with one-to-one assistance from the teacher when necessary. Daily computer-assisted drills were also required. Direct observations of David during independent seatwork conditions indicated that he was off-task for approximately 25% of the observed intervals. Similar data collected while he was engaged in computer-assisted drills showed he was off-task for only 14% of the observed intervals.

Teacher Consultation

After discussing the results of the initial assessment with his teacher and other classroom personnel, it was agreed that an intervention would be implemented, which was designed to increase the pace of moving through material and thus narrow the three-grade discrepancy between David's current functioning and the expected grade placement based on his chronological age. After reviewing several options, the consultation team decided to use a self-management spelling intervention incorporating audiotaped drill sessions. Words from the first eight units of the new spelling book (15 words per unit) were targeted for learning. The long-term objectives for a 7-week intervention program were to:

1. Attain 85% of the mean possible letter sequences correct on probes that randomly incorporate words from the eight targeted units.
2. Spell 14 of 17 words correctly from these same probes.

Self-Managing Spelling Intervention

The full details of this procedure were described in Chapter 3, and will only be summarized here. Two word lists on audiotapes were prepared for each unit. The first list, the practice list, was generated by saying the first word, waiting 7–10 seconds, spelling the word, and then repeating this sequence for each of the 15 words on the list. The second tape, the test tape, was generated in a similar fashion, excluding the spelling of the words. Step-by-step written directions for both practice and test sessions were also provided for David.

During practice sessions, David was given a prepared sheet of paper and the tape. For each taped word, David was taught to listen to the word, place the recorder on pause, write the word, turn the recorder back on, and then write the word again as the word was spelled on the tape. David was instructed to compare his spelling with the tape's spelling. If the two matched, he was told to move on to the next word. If the two did not match, he was told to place the recorder on pause again and write the word correctly three times in the space provided. At the end of the session, David used an "Easy Grader" device to calculate the percentage of words that were correct on his first attempt. Once computed, he graphed the results.

If David earned 100% on any given practice session, he was eligible to take a test on the entire unit. The procedures of the test follow those described above, except that the words are not spelled on the tape. After completing the test, David was instructed to refer back to the practice sheet where he had scored 100% to evaluate his test performance. He then graded and graphed his test results. If his test performance was 85% or better, David was permitted to move to the next unit. If his performance was less than 85%, he was required to continue practice sessions on that unit.

The practice and/or test sessions were held once per day. In addition, David completed daily computer-assisted drills as he had before the implementation of the sessions. The teacher also required the completion of related spelling assignments for each unit using self-management techniques. These required him to write each word three times, write complete sentences using each word, alphabetize all the words in a unit, and write definitions for each word using a dictionary. He was not required to fully complete the related assignments in order to move to the next unit if he met the 100% practice and 85% test criteria.

To motivate David to comply with the self-management program, he was provided with one comic book each time he received a score of 100% on a test after spending a maximum of 4 days on that unit. David was given the responsibility for informing the teacher when he had achieved the criterion.

Twice each week, a curriculum-based measurement (CBM) probe of spelling was administered. These probes involved selecting 2 to 3 words randomly from each of the eight units to generate a total of 20 words per CBM probe. The words were dictated every 7 seconds during a 2-minute period. If David completed a word prior to the 7-second time frame, another word was dictated. The results of these probes were scored and graphed by the teacher using the CBM procedure of correct letters in a sequence per minute (see Shapiro, 1989b for more details on this scoring procedure) and total correct words spelled. The results were shared with David each week.

Results

Figures 7.1 and 7.2 show the results of the administration of the CBM probes. Average performance during baseline was 35 letter sequences correct and 4.6 words spelled correctly. Goals for the 7-week intervention were set at 45.5 letter sequences correct and 14 words spelled correctly. As shown by the data, David made remarkable progress in the 7-week period, clearly moving toward his goal on both metrics.

The results of David's practice and test performance are shown Figure 7.3. Clear evidence of learning across days was

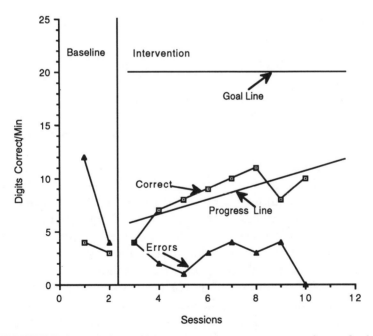

FIGURE 7.1. Number of letter sequences correct per minute during each assessment session with David.

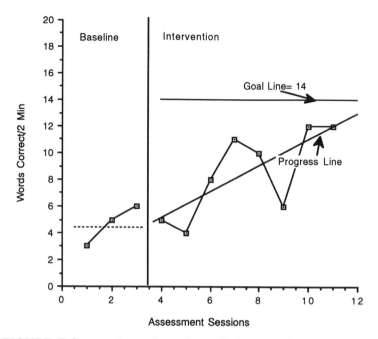

FIGURE 7.2. Number of words spelled correctly per 2 minutes during each assessment session with David.

present from the results of the practice sessions, where the number of days to reach 100% on the practice lists ranged from 2 to 4 days. On all tests, David achieved 100% performance.

David indicated great satisfaction in using the newly learned self-management spelling procedure. He stated that he enjoyed learning to spell using procedures very different from those accompanying the typical workbook activities. The incorporation of procedures such as writing sentences, arranging words in alphabetical order, and looking up definitions, in addition to the taped drill procedure, facilitated learning beyond the rote drill of spelling words out of context. Additionally, David indicated that he was very aware of his progress because of the self-graphing procedure. He was encouraged by his teacher to explain the procedure to peers.

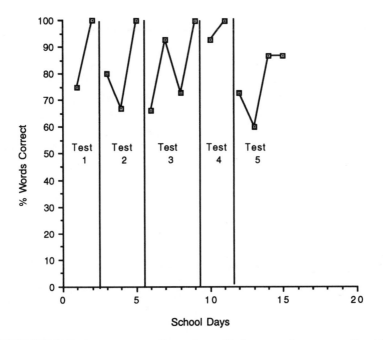

FIGURE 7.3. Percentage of words spelled correctly on tests David took each school day.

Comments

This case illustrates how the self-managed spelling procedure described in Chapter 3 can be easily implemented in a classroom setting to address a difficult problem, which many children struggle with academically. Typically, teachers are frustrated because the slow pace of progress made by these children means they require greater attention than their peers do. The teacher often has great difficulty finding the time to provide individualized instruction that will supplement the existing instructional procedures. Yet with this case, the procedure was implemented with very little need for teacher monitoring or evaluation.

In this case illustration, a student who was currently at a level several grades below expectation was provided with a procedure that could easily accelerate his progress through curriculum materials. At the same time, the procedure ensured that he learned more than the spelling of the words, since he also engaged in activities teachers would find highly acceptable such as writing sentences, alphabetizing words, and looking up dictionary definitions. The results of the intervention for David provided an opportunity to experience success at a level he rarely had experienced in school. Indeed, having him explain the procedure to his peers was probably another very motivating experience. Hence, the student was likely to learn self-management skills beyond the scope of the spelling lessons.

Case 2: Paul—Self-Monitoring Math Performance

Background

Paul was a 15-year-old boy who was attending a self-contained program for children with SED. At the time this intervention was conducted, he was in a combined 7th–8th grade classroom situated in a local school district. Paul had been placed in the classroom for children with SED almost 4 years previous to the intervention. At that time his behavior was reported to be extremely aggressive, noncompliant, and out of control. Over the last year, Paul had become increasingly disruptive around the completion of his math assignments, consistently claiming that the assigned math was "too hard."

Initial Assessment and Teacher Consultation

Through an interview with Paul's teacher, it was learned that the assignments were well within Paul's instructional level. This was confirmed by examining some of Paul's completed worksheets. Prior to beginning the intervention, baseline data collected over a 5-day period showed that Paul was accurately completing an average of only 9.4 problems per day during a 40-minute math class. More importantly, the data showed a steady decline over the week to a low of only six problems completed during the math classes. According to his teacher, students were expected to complete approximately 15 problems per week.

In consultation with Paul's teacher, it was decided that Paul needed to become more aware of his completion rates during math periods. In addition, it was hoped that increasing his math performance would subsequently reduce the amount of off-task, out-of-seat, and other disruptive behaviors that he was displaying during math class. To accomplish this goal, the consultation team decided to implement a self-monitoring program.

A Self-Monitoring Math Intervention

Paul was given a recording sheet with three columns, including the date, the number of problems completed, and the number of problems completed correctly. He was instructed that at the end of each math class, he was to have his paper corrected by the teacher or the classroom aide and then record the information in the appropriate columns. Paul was also taught how to graph his performance.

In order to provide effective motivation, Paul was allowed to select a potential reward for meeting a preset criterion for performance (15 problems correct per day). Paul chose to work toward a particular cassette tape. For each day he met the criterion, he would earn $.50 toward the purchase of the tape. On certain days, he could also earn extra money for completing more than the required 15 problems. However, Paul would not be informed whether the day was a bonus day until after the math period had ended. Paul was also able to earn an additional $1.00 toward the tape purchase if he maintained an entire week at or above the 15-problem criterion.

All procedures were reviewed with Paul and a contract was signed between Paul, the teacher, and the school psychologist who had helped develop the intervention (see Figure, 7.4). Throughout the intervention, Paul's recording sheet was checked periodically to ensure its accuracy.

Contract

1. **Every day I will keep track of the number of problems I complete during math. There are two steps to this procedure:**

   A) fill out the ditto sheet;
   B) mark number of problems correct on graph.

2. **Each day I accurately complete the number of problems or more indicated by the dark line I will earn fifty cents, which Miss Kates will keep for me so I can earn a tape: BIG DADDY KANE!! Certain days may be "bonus days" in which I can earn extra money. I need to earn $8.00 to buy the tape. If I have an entire week above the goal line, I can earn an extra dollar.**

I agree to the steps outlines in this contract.

   3/27/90   **Paul**

   3/27/90   **Miss Kates**

FIGURE 7.4. Behavioral contract for Paul.

Results

Figure 7.5 shows the results of the self-monitoring intervention over the 3 weeks of the intervention. During the first week of the intervention, Paul completed an average of 10 problems correct per day. In addition, his performance declined over the week. However, during the second week, Paul's performance showed a dramatic improvement, where he averaged 16 problems correct per day. This level of performance was maintained during the third and final week of implementation. Over the period of implementation, Paul earned $5.00 toward the tape and was treated to lunch by the school psychologist. Unfortunately, the intervention had to be discontinued prior to Paul's earning the cassette tape since he had begun to be mainstreamed for all of his classes and was moved to another building.

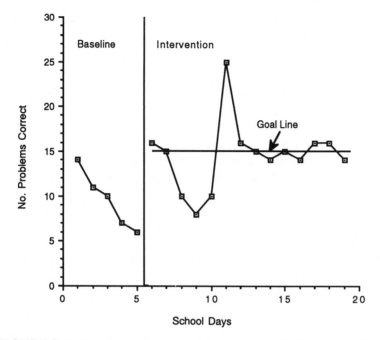

FIGURE 7.5. Number of math problems correct during each school day for Paul.

Discussion

This case illustrates the potential ease of using self-monitoring procedures with an adolescent. In this case, the problem was first identified as a "won't-do" rather than a "can't-do" problem. Such distinctions are quite important since it would be unreasonable to expect a self-monitoring program aimed at accurate performance to be effective if the student is unable to accurately perform the work. In Paul's case, the intervention may have been effective since it was already known that Paul was capable of doing the assignments.

A particularly important component of this intervention might have been the presence of the reward. While the case study does not allow one to know if self-monitoring alone would have been effective, it is important to note that the inclusion of rewards are not always necessary to obtain the desired results. However, when working with students who have a history of disruptive behavior as well as academic problems, inclusion of rewards within self-management programs is probably highly desirable. In conclusion, the case of Paul clearly demonstrates the ease with which a self-monitoring type of program can be implemented. The technique required very little teacher monitoring or input and resulted in highly effective outcomes.

Case 3: Vincent—Self-Monitoring Homework Assignments

Background

Vincent was an 11-year-old boy who currently attended the sixth grade of a middle school. Vincent was referred by his teachers due to their concerns regarding his lack of motivation, failure to complete homework assignments, and difficulties remaining focused throughout activities during the day. Among these problems, assignment completion, especially homework was found to be the most troublesome to his teachers. At the time of this intervention, Vincent attended a resource room for children with learning disabilities approximately 2 hours per day.

Initial Assessment

Vincent's teachers estimated that he had been completing only about 5% of his daily homework assignments. In addition, Vincent's teachers reported that he frequently engaged in off-task behaviors, including tapping pencils, looking around the room, talking with nearby students, drawing, and daydreaming. Enacting consequences for these behaviors, such as removing points from Vincent that were part of a classwide token economy system during the resource room, as well as verbal reprimands, had been ineffective.

Baseline data included collecting both the percentage of assignments completed per day and direct observation of Vincent's on-task behavior. Over three observations made in one classroom over several days lasting approximately 30 minutes each, Vincent was found to be off-task for the observed intervals in comparison to peers who averaged only 10% off-task behavior during the same time. The number of completed homework assignments over an 8-day period were calculated. On the first 3 days, Vincent completed all assignments (1 or 2 per night), but then failed to complete all but one assignment over the last 5 days of data collection (usually 2 to 3 were assigned per night).

Teacher Consultation

In meeting with Vincent's teachers it was noted that, although Vincent always took the appropriate books home each evening, he failed to do his homework most nights. The teachers reported that the data from the last 5 days of baseline were more typical of Vincent than the initial 3 days, during which he completed the assignments. In discussing Vincent's failure to complete homework, his teachers indicated that all assignments were based on current instructional levels and well within his academic capacity.

During a meeting with the school psychologist, a series of potential interventions were discussed. It was decided to implement a self-monitoring procedure to potentially motivate Vincent to complete his homework assignments. The entire procedure would be monitored by the resource room teacher, but would include homework from across his various subjects. To provide additional motivation, Vincent would be able to earn a selected reward to be shared with the entire resource room class if he met his goal. An initial goal was set that would require Vincent to complete two of three assignments per night, and 80% of assignments per week to be eligible for the weekly reward.

Self-Monitoring for Homework Assignment Completion

A self-monitoring chart was generated and taped to Vincent's desk (see Figure 7.6). Each morning, Vincent would record whether or not he had completed the homework by writing a "Yes" or "No" in the corresponding square. In addition, his weekly reward was written on the chart.

	Monday	Tuesday	Wednesday	Thursday	Friday
Journal					
Spelling					
Reading					
English					
Social Studies					
Math					

Goal I am working for this week:

1. Each morning check the chart.

2. For each subject write:

   Yes- If you finished your work

   No- If you did not finish your work

   X- If you had no homework in that subject

This week ___ assignments must be completed to earn goal.

FIGURE 7.6. Vincent's self-monitoring chart for the completion of homework assignments.

Results

Figure 7.7 shows the results of the intervention. Each night, Vincent received between one and five assignments. As soon as the intervention was implemented, he immediately began to complete all the assignments, and maintained this level of performance throughout the 11 days of the intervention.

Clearly, the intervention was highly effective. Vincent began to complete almost all of his work and soon improved his grades in all of his academic subjects as well. A particularly interesting side effect of the intervention was the gains in social skills that emerged when Vincent began earning weekly rewards for the entire class.

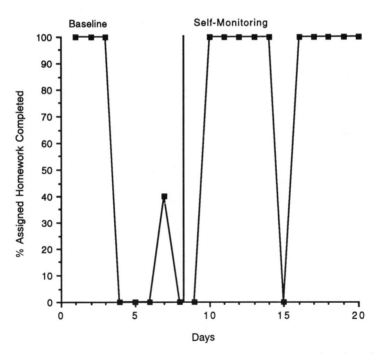

FIGURE 7.7. Number of homework assignments completed each school day by Vincent.

Comments

This was a rather simple but powerful intervention. Very simply, the student checked each morning to see if he had completed his homework. It also offered an easy method for the teacher to impact an area of difficulty that had been very problematic for this student. In addition, the procedure described was applied across all academic subject areas without difficulty.

An interesting feature of this case study was the use of the resource room teacher as the source for implementation and monitoring of the self-management intervention. Often, when children experience problems and are in the middle school or high school, it is quite difficult to involve all teachers in an intervention program. By using the resource room teacher as the program implementor, it was possible to impact Vincent's behavior across all subjects without directly involving any of his other teachers. It is highly recommended that, when using interventions of this type at the middle- or high-school levels, a specific individual be responsible for monitoring the overall program (e.g., guidance counselor, school psychologist, special education teacher). Such an arrangement makes conducting this form of self-management very feasible for students who have multiple teachers.

As in the previous case, it is important that interventions aimed at improving performance do not ask students to perform tasks that are outside of their capability. The use of such tasks would likely have detrimental effects on the student since he or she might not successfully complete the work because he or she was not able to do it, not because of lack of motivation.

Case 4: Colin—Self-Monitoring of Math Performance

Background

Colin was a second-grade student who was having significant problems with the mastery of basic math facts. While he was currently functioning at grade level in reading and spelling, he was at approximately a first-grade level in math. All of his instruction occurred within the regular classroom.

Initial Assessment

At the time of the assessment, Colin was being instructed in the second-grade book of the math series. Not surprisingly, he was struggling with this level of material. Math was taught to the entire class (approximately 25 students) during a daily 45-minute period, of which about 30 minutes was allocated for individual seatwork. According to his teacher, Colin had not yet mastered basic addition and subtraction facts and counted on his fingers even for simple problems. His teacher had tried to move him forward with the rest of the class and had been helping him with regrouping from the ones to the tens column in addition and subtraction.

A curriculum-based assessment of math showed that Colin had mastered addition problems with sums to 10, and was instructional for sums of 11 to 19. In subtraction, he performed at a frustrational level when adding numbers that summed up to 18 and did not understand the algorithm for subtracting 1-digit numbers from a 2-digit number when the answer was less than 18.

Self-Monitoring of Math Facts: Cover, Copy, and Compare

After consulting with Colin's teacher, it was decided to teach Colin a method for self-monitoring his math computation skills during a specific drill activity. A procedure called "Cover, Copy, and Compare" (CCC) described by Skinner et al. (1989), was used with addition and subtraction facts. The steps in the procedure were as follows:

1. At least three times per week Colin was given two worksheets with a list of 10 problems each (one sheet of addition and one of subtraction). The complete problems with their answers were provided on the sheets.
2. On each sheet, Colin was trained to first look at the problem, then cover it with an index card, and write the problem twice in the space provided next to the original problem.

3. Colin would then uncover the original problem and check to see if his answers were correct. If not, he was to write the problem again.

4. Following his drill, Colin was given a CBM probe containing 30 problems, which were randomly selected from 1-digit minus 2-digit subtraction problems that were not regrouped, and 1-digit addition problems with sums from 11–19. Colin was given 2 minutes to complete as many of these as he could. He was then given an answer sheet so that he could check his responses, and graph the total number of problems correct.

Results of Colin's performance are shown in Figure 7.8. As can be seen, Colin showed steady improvement toward mastery of his computational skills.

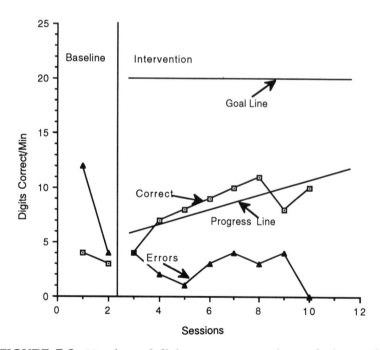

FIGURE 7.8. Number of digits correct per minute during each session with Colin.

Comments

The results of this simple and easily implemented self-management procedure show how self-generated practice and drill exercises can significantly improve the performance of a child struggling with an academic area. Of particular note is the fact that the procedure allowed Colin to begin to make up lost ground within the regular classroom. Because of this, he was able to be taught with the rest of the class.

NONACADEMIC SKILLS PROBLEMS

Case 5: Michael—Self-Monitoring Transitions between Academic Subjects

Background

Michael was a seventh-grade student (age 12 years), who was enrolled in a self-contained classroom for students with behavior disorders. He was referred to the school psychologist because he consistently caused problems whenever the teacher needed to switch to a new academic subject. Specifically, each time the teacher changed academic tasks, Michael needed repeated verbal reminders to gather the appropriate materials, sit in his seat, and begin the new assignment.

Initial Assessment and Teacher Consultation

In consultation with the teacher, three specific behaviors were defined as necessary to establish good transition skills: gathering all required materials for the next class activity, seating oneself in the appropriate area, and engaging in these without other inappropriate behavior.

Data were collected by the teacher, who recorded whether or not, in his judgment, Michael had engaged in appropriate transition behavior at each point in the school day between 9:00 A.M. and 2:45 P.M. when a new academic task was introduced. Over a 5-day period, Michael engaged in appropriate transitions approximately 64% of the time.

Self-Monitoring: Academic Transition Behavior

Based on the teacher's data, a self-monitoring intervention was planned. Data sheets were generated by having Michael help design a recording sheet. Next to a drawing of an eagle, the following list of transition rules were provided:

1. Gather all materials.
2. Sit in appropriate area.
3. Do these quickly and quietly.

Below these rules were directions instructing Michael to mark a plus sign (+) if the transition rules were followed appropriately, and a minus sign (−) if they were not. The remainder of the data sheet consisted of a grid for recording these responses (see Figure 7.9). The grid had 35 boxes arranged in five columns, labeled as days of the week, and seven rows, labeled with each of the seven academic periods of the day.

Before beginning the procedure each day, Michael was permitted to select tokens from a reinforcement menu which he could earn contingent on completing 100% of the transitions appropriately. At the same time as Michael did, the teacher also judged Michael's behavior. However, Michael was rewarded on the basis of the data collected, not that collected by his teacher.

Results

Figure 7.10 shows the impact of the intervention. Over the 10 days of the intervention, Michael showed a dramatic and substantial increase in his level of appropriate transitions per day. These data reflect actual performance, as rated by Michael. When compared to the data collected by the teacher, Michael was accurate 93% of the time, suggesting that he was fairly honest about recording inappropriate transitions when they occurred.

At the end of the 10 days of the intervention, the requirements for recording transition behavior were faded, so that Michael only collected data twice, and then once, per week.

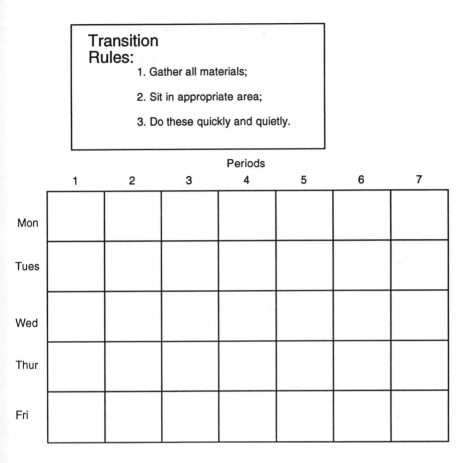

FIGURE 7.9. Michael's self-monitoring sheet for transition behavior.

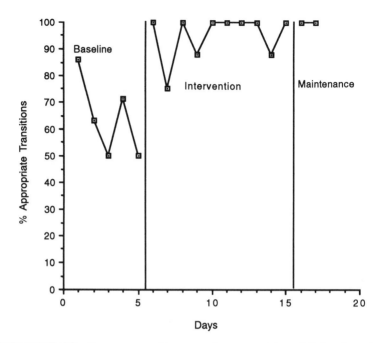

FIGURE 7.10. Percentage of appropriate transitions Michael made during each school day.

Michael maintained 100% appropriate transition behavior during this time.

Comments

The simple procedure of having Michael self-monitor the presence of a series of specific behaviors required for appropriate transition, along with providing a backup reward, was highly successful in improving his behavior. Although contingent rewards were included, Michael was responsible for generating his own list of them, selecting a reward when appropriate, and approaching the teacher to communicate his choice. Additionally, the reward was provided at the end of the school day and was thus removed in time from many of the appropriate transitions that he made. While there is some evidence in the literature that self-monitoring without a contingent reward can be effective, other research has shown that self-monitoring combined with a reward is a more powerful combination. This combination, was specifically requested by Michael's teachers.

Case 6: Carrie—Self-Monitoring and Habit Reversal for Thumb Sucking

Background

Carrie was an 8-year-old girl in the second grade who was observed by her teacher to often have long periods of time when she would suck her thumb during class. The occasional ridicule and teasing Carrie would receive from her peers was clearly of great concern. At the time of this intervention, Carrie had been referred for possible placement in a classroom for children with emotional disturbance.

Initial Assessment

Data were collected by counting the number of instances in which Carrie sucked her thumb during two 1-hour periods over a 10-day interval. The first hour was observed during a math class and the second hour during a science/social studies class. Each time Carrie removed her thumb an instance was counted. Results showed that she averaged 7.9 instances of thumb sucking between the two 1-hour periods each day. Clearly, this was a significant and substantially high frequency problem.

Self-Monitoring and Habit Reversal

After consulting with the teacher, two sets of procedures were simultaneously implemented. A habit-reversal technique known to help reduce thumb-sucking behavior was first taught to Carrie. This procedure involved having her clench her fist with the thumb inside her hand whenever she felt the urge to suck her thumb. In addition, a self-monitoring procedure was generated. Carrie was given a self-monitoring sheet divided

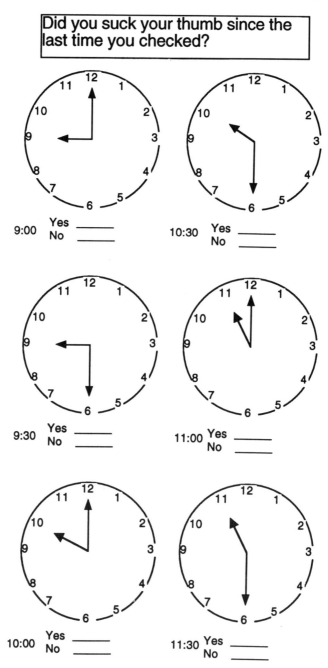

FIGURE 7.11. Carrie's self-monitoring sheet for thumb sucking.

into 30-minute intervals (see Figure 7.11). This sheet also contained clocks, which indicated the time at these intervals. Carrie was instructed to mark a "Yes" or "No" every 30 minutes based on whether she had kept her thumb out of her mouth during that interval. A daily criteria of 75% (9 out of 12) intervals without thumb sucking was set for Carrie to earn a chosen reward.

Results

Figure 7.12 shows the results of the intervention. Carrie reduced her frequency of thumbsucking (as collected at the same 2-hour period as in baseline) from a mean of 7.9 instances per day to 0.3 occurrences. This reduction was substantial and resulted in reported improvements in peer relationships as well.

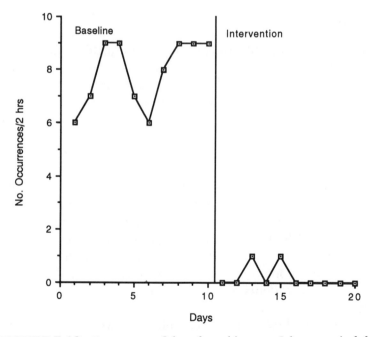

FIGURE 7.12. Frequency of thumb sucking per 2-hour period during each school day for Carrie.

Comments

The problem in this intervention is often a difficult one to tackle. Habits are often very problematic to disrupt and can lead to significantly stigmatizing outcomes for children. The combination of self-monitoring and habit reversal, along with contingent reward for performance, worked together to successfully reduce Carrie's thumbsucking. More importantly, the intervention was done in the context of a regular classroom environment without any substantial investment of teacher time. Again, the use of self-management shows the potential of significant improvement in student behavior problems by placing the behavior under the control of the student him- or herself.

Case 7: Alice— Social Skills Training for a Socially Withdrawn Child

Background

Alice was a 6-year-old girl enrolled in a regular, half-day kindergarten program. She was functioning at an age-appropriate academic level, but rarely initiated interactions with peers and preferred to play alone. At the time this intervention was implemented, school staff was considering whether Alice needed special educational programming for emotional support.

Initial Assessment

To determine the specific behaviors to target for social skills training, the Social Skills Rating Scale (SSRS, Gresham & Elliott, 1990) was administered to Alice's teacher. Using the results of the SSRS, Alice's teacher was asked to further describe the primary behavior problems that were indicated on the measure. Additionally, the teacher was asked to indicate behaviors which students did not exhibit but were critical social skills in their classrooms.

Based on these data, three behaviors were targeted for Alice. These were operationally defined as:

1. *Initiates conversation with peers*—a verbal statement or question addressed to a peer that resulted in a response from that peer. This definition did not include statements made to the teacher or aide, requests for objects, calling out, or responses to words initiated by a peer.

2. *Gives compliments to peers*—a verbal statement to a peer that conveyed praise of behavior, appearance, or material possessions. This definition did not include compliments to the teacher or aide.

3. *Invites others to join in an activity*—a verbal statement or question to a peer(s) to join in a free-time activity. Statements may have been in the form of asking a peer to join the target student or asking the peer if the target student can join the peer(s).

Social Skills Training

Using direct, systematic observation, data were obtained in the regular classroom environment on the frequency of the occurrence of these behaviors during an art/free-time period. After baseline was completed, social skills training was provided to Alice in a group of three students twice a week for 30-minute sessions. After each training session, observational data were again collected in the art/free-time period.

The social skills training program used was a multimethod training package designed to facilitate transfer of skills to the regular classroom. Specifically, the procedure incorporated the following techniques:

1. *Instructions*: Sessions began with a discussion about why a particular skill was important, when the skill should be used, and how to perform the skill. Students were requested to respond to questions asked by the trainer. Many examples of the skill being taught were recited. For example, with the skill "complimenting," the trainer explained that complimenting referred to saying nice things to others that make them feel happy. Alice and the other children were then asked for ex-

amples of "complimenting" that they had done or seen others do.

2. *Modeling*: The trainer modeled performance of the skill with all of the children. Multiple response exemplars were used. Continuing with the example of "complimenting," the trainer instructed one of the children to be a confederate and pretend to give a complement to the trainer. Each participant had a chance to be the confederate. For instance, the confederate might be told to say to the trainer, "I got these new sneakers for Christmas." The trainer would then model a response such as, "Those are the neatest sneakers I've ever seen."

3. *Behavior rehearsal*: Each student in the group was then given five opportunities to demonstrate a skill with another peer. The trainer would provide prompts such as, "Alice, I'd like you to show everyone what you would do if you wanted to join Tom in playing a game." Both students were prompted to respond.

4. *Feedback*: Students were provided feedback regarding the accuracy of the rehearsals by each peer involved in the interaction. For example, after a role play was completed, the trainer might say, "Alice, please tell Tom if he did a good job of explaining the rules. Should he have done anything differently?" The trainer then modeled and had the children practice how to give appropriate feedback.

5. *Praise*: Descriptive praise was provided for each student for accurate performance throughout the training.

In addition to providing social skills training, specific efforts were made by Alice's classroom teacher to facilitate her using the skills in the regular classroom setting. Specifically, a training chart was made with all of the students names and drawings relating to the skills to be trained. This was placed in the front of Alice's classroom. Second, Alice was prompted to tell her teacher, aide, and her peers when she had performed one of the skills or observed a peer performing one of the skills. Third, the teacher placed a sticker next to Alice's name anytime she was observed engaging in the behavior in the classroom. Finally, Alice was permitted to select a desired reward if she used at least one skill during the art/free-play period.

Results

Figure 7.13 shows the results of social skills training on Alice's performance during the art/free-play period. With the beginning of training, Alice showed a substancial increase in all three skills. All behaviors showed good maintenance after training was concluded, although some decline in joining was observed.

Comments

Clearly, the implementation of social skills training resulted in excellent improvements in Alice's targeted behaviors. Of particular impressiveness, the social skills training showed good generalization effects from the training session, which was done outside the classroom, to actual behavioral responses in the classroom. This was most likely due to the presence of several programmed procedures designed to facilitate generalization. Indeed, because social skills training rarely results in the transfer of skills from the training to nontraining settings, it is crucial that efforts be made to provide antecedents and consequences that will likely elicit the learned social behaviors in settings different from where the behavior was trained.

FINAL COMMENTS

Throughout this and other chapters, we have presented example after example of how self-management procedures can be applied to school-based problems. The simplicity with which self-management can be done has been consistently shown with these examples. Given the ease of using such procedures, we question why they have not been employed more often by teachers.

Hopefully, the material presented, both in the form of case studies and research, provides rich and substantial data

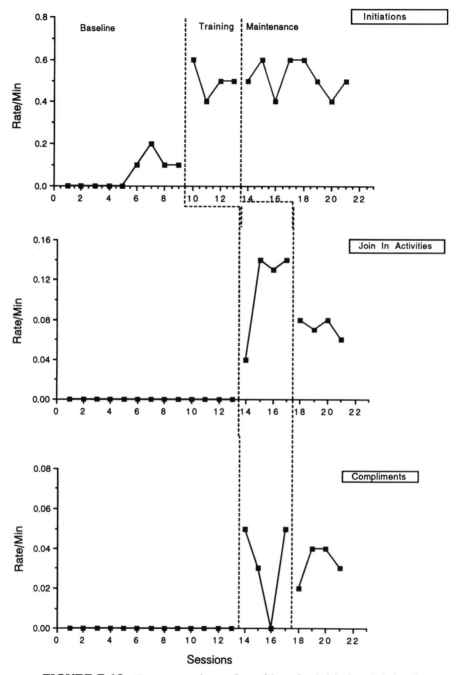

FIGURE 7.13. Rate per minute for taking the initiative, joining in activities, and delivering compliments during daily sessions for Alice.

upon which practice can be based. There is little question that self-management is the goal for every teacher in working with every student. Although self-management does not always emerge on its own, there certainly is an extensive technology for teaching these skills. We sincerely believe that the increased use of these procedures will lead to better academic, social, and emotional performance among students. We also believe that the use of self-management procedures is likely to improve a student's self-concept and feelings of self-worth. Further, we doubt that psychologists, teachers, or other school personnel exist who do not wish the same for all the students they touch. While certainly not a panacea for solving all of the problems faced by teachers in school, self-management procedures offer opportunities to establish long-term changes among students who are struggling with academic or nonacademic problems.

References

Ager, C. L., & Cole, C. L. (1991). A review of cognitive–behavioral interventions for children and adolescents with behavioral disorders. *Behavioral Disorders, 16*, 276–287.

Agran, M., Fodor-Davis, J., Moore, S., & Deer, M. (1989). The application of a self-management program on instruction-following skills. *Journal of the Association for Persons with Severe Handicaps, 14*, 147–154.

Agran, M., Salzberg, C. L., & Stowitschek, J. J. (1987). An analysis of the effects of a social skills training program using self-instruction on the acquisition and generalization of two social behaviors in a work setting. *Journal of the Association for Persons with Severe Handicaps, 12*, 131–139.

Alberto, P. A., Sharpton, W. R., Briggs, A. H., & Stright, M. H. (1986). Facilitating task acquisition through the use of a self-operated auditory prompting system. *Journal of the Association for Persons with Severe Handicaps, 11*, 85–91.

Alessi, G. (1988). Direct observation methods for emotional/behavior problems. In E. S. Shapiro & T. R. Kratochwill (Eds.), *Behavioral assessment in schools: Conceptual foundations and practical applications* (pp. 14–75). New York: Guilford Press.

Amabile, T. M., & Gitomer, J. (1984). Children's artistic creativity: Effects of choice in task materials. *Personality & Social Psychology Bulletin, 10*, 209–215.

Bambara, L. M., & Ager, C. (1992). Using self-scheduling to promote self-directed leisure activity in home and community settings. *Journal of the Association for Persons with Severe Handicaps, 17*, 67–76.

Bandura, A. (1976). Self-reinforcement: Theoretical and methodological considerations. *Behaviorism, 4*, 135–155.

Bannerman, D. J., Sheldon, J. B., Sherman, J. A., & Harchik, A. E. (1990). Balancing the right to habilitation with the right to personal liberties:

The rights of people with developmental disabilities to eat too many doughnuts and take a nap. *Journal of Applied Behavior Analysis, 23*, 79–89.

Bash, M. A., & Camp, B. W. (1986). Teacher training in the Think Aloud program. In G. Cartledge & J. F. Milburn (Eds.), *Teaching social skills to children: Innovative approaches* (2nd ed., pp. 187–218). New York: Pergamon Press.

Baumgart, D., Brown, L., Pumpian, I., Nisbet, J., Ford, A., Sweet, M., Messina, R., & Schroeder, J. (1982). Principle of partial participation and individualized adaptations in educational programs for severely handicapped students. *Journal of the Association for the Severely Handicapped, 7*, 17–27.

Beck, A. (1963). Thinking and depression: 1. Idiosyncratic content and cognitive distortions. *Archives of General Psychiatry, 9*, 324–333.

Beck, A. T., Rush, A. J., Shaw, B. E., & Emery, G. (1979). *Cognitive therapy of depression.* New York: Guilford Press.

Billings, D. C., & Wasik, B. H. (1985). Self-instructional training with preschoolers: An attempt to replicate. *Journal of Applied Behavior Analysis, 18*, 61–67.

Bird, F., Dores, P. A., Moniz, D., & Robinson, J. (1989). Reducing severe aggressive and self-injuriuos behaviors with functional communication training. *American Journal on Mental Retardation, 94*, 37–48.

Bornstein, P., & Quevillon, R. (1976). Modifications of severe disruptive and aggressive behavior using brief timeout and reinforcement procedures. *Journal of Applied Behavior Analysis, 2*, 21–38.

Brigham, T. A. (1979). Some effects of choice on academic performance. In L. C. Perlmuter & R. A. Monty (Eds.), *Choice and perceived control* (pp. 131–142). Hillsdale, NJ: Erlbaum.

Brigham, T. A. (1989). *Self-management for adolescents: A skills training program.* New York: Guilford Press.

Broden, M., Hall, R. V., & Mitts, B. (1971). The effects of self-recording on the classroom behavior of two eighth grade students. *Journal of Applied Behavior Analysis, 4*, 191–199.

Browder, D. M., & Shapiro, E. S. (1985). Applications of self-management to individuals with severe handicaps: A review. *Journal of the Association for Persons with Severe Handicaps, 10*, 200–208.

Bryant, L. I., & Budd, K. S. (1982). Self-instructional training to increase independent work performance in preschoolers. *Journal of Applied Behavior Analysis, 15*, 259–271.

Burgio, L. D., Whitman, T. L., & Johnson, M. R. (1980). A self-instructional package for increasing attending behavior in educable mentally retarded children. *Journal of Applied Behavior Analysis, 13*, 443–459.

Buyer, L. S., Berkson, G., Winnega, M. A., & Morton, L. (1987). Stimulation and control as components of stereotyped body rocking. *American Journal of Mental Deficiency, 91*, 543–547.

Camp, B. W., & Bash, M. S. (1985a). *Think Aloud: Increasing social and cog-*

nitive skills—A problem-solving program for children, Classroom program grades 1–2. Champaign, IL: Research Press.

Camp, B. W., & Bash, M. S. (1985b). *Think Aloud: Increasing social and cognitive skills—A problem-solving program for children. Classroom program grades 3–4*. Champaign, IL: Research Press.

Camp, B. W., & Bash, M. S. (1985c). *Think Aloud: Increasing social and cognitive skills—A problem-solving program for children, Classroom program grades 5–6*. Champaign, IL: Research Press.

Camp, B. W., Blom, G. E., Hebert, F., & Van Doorninck, W. J. (1977). "Think aloud": A program for developing self-control in young aggressive boys. *Journal of Abnormal Child Psychology, 5*, 157–169.

Carr, E. G., & Durand, V. M (1985). Reducing problem behaviors through functional communication training. *Journal of Applied Behavior Analysis, 18*, 111–126.

Carr, E. G., & Newsom, C. (1985). Demand-related tantrums: Conceptualization and treatment. *Behavior Modification, 9*, 403–426.

Carr, E. G., Newsom, C. D., & Binkhoff, J. A. (1980). Escape as a factor in the aggressive behavior of two retarded children. *Journal of Applied Behavior Analysis, 13*, 101–117.

Charlop, M. H., Burgio, L. D., Iwata, B. A., & Ivancic, M. T. (1988). Stimulus variation as a means of enhancing punishment effects. *Journal of Applied Behavior Analysis, 21*, 89–93.

Christie, D. J., Hiss, M., & Lozanoff, B. (1984). Modification of inattentive classroom behavior: Hyperactive children's use of self-recording with teacher guidance. *Behavior Modification, 8*, 391–406.

Clark, E., Kehle, T. J., Jenson, W. R., & Beck, D. E. (1992). Evaluation of the parameters of self-modeling interventions. *School Psychology Review, 21*, 246–254.

Cole, C. L., & Bambara, L. M. (1992). Issues surrounding the use of self-management interventions in the schools. *School Psychology Review, 21*, 193–201.

Craighead, W. E., Wilcoxon-Craighead, L., & Meyers, A. W. (1978). New directions in behavior modification with children. In M. Hersen, R. M. Eisler, & P. M. Miller (Eds.), *Progress in behavior modification* (Vol. 6, pp. 159–201). New York: Academic Press.

Dattilo, J., & Rusch, F. R. (1985). Effects of choice on leisure participation for persons with severe handicaps. *Journal of the Association for Persons with Severe Handicaps, 10*, 194–199.

Deffenbacher, J. L & Suinn, R. M. (1982). The self-control of anxiety. In P. Karoly & F. H. Kanfer (Eds.), *Self-management and behavior change: From theory to practice* (pp. 393–442). New York: Pergamon Press.

Deshler, D. D., & Schumaker, J. B. (1988). An instructional model for teaching students how to learn. In J. L. Graden, J. E. Zins, & M. J. Curtis (Eds.)., *Alternative educational delivery systems: Enhancing instructional options for all students* (pp. 391–411). Washington, DC: National Assocation of School Psychologists.

DiGangi, S. A., Maag, J. W., & Rutherford, R. B. Jr. (1991). Self-graphing of on-task behavior: Enhancing the reactive effects of self-monitoring on on-task behavior and academic performance. *Learning Disabilities Quarterly, 14*, 221–230.

Dowrick, P. W., & Dove, C. (1980). The use of self-modeling to improve the swimming performance of spina bifida children. *Journal of Applied Behavior Analysis, 13*, 51–56.

Dunlap, L. K., & Dunlap, G. (1989). A self-monitoring package for teaching subtraction with regrouping to students with learning disabilities. *Journal of Applied Behavior Analysis, 22*, 309–314.

Dush, D. M., Hirt, M. L., & Schroeder, H. E. (1989). Self-statement modification in the treatment of child behavior disorders: A meta-analysis. *Psychological Bulletin, 106*, 97–106.

Dyer, K. (1987). The competition of autistic stereotyped behavior with usual and specially assessed reinforcers. *Research in Developmental Disabilities, 8*, 607–626.

Dyer, K., Dunlap, G., & Winterling, V. (1989, May). The effects of choice-making on the problem behaviors of students with severe disabilities. In G. Dunlap (Chair), *Community-referenced research on behavior management*. Symposium conducted at the fifteenth annual convention of the Association for Behavior Analysis, Milwaukee, WI.

Dyer, K., Dunlap, G., & Winterling, V. (1990). Effects of choice making on the serious problem behaviors of students with severe handicaps. *Journal of Applied Behavior Analysis, 23*, 515–524.

D'Zurilla, T. J., & Goldfried, M. R. (1971). Problem solving and behavior modification. *Journal of Abnormal Psychology, 78*, 107–126.

Erin, J. N., Dignan, K., & Brown, P. A. (1991). Are social skills teachable? A review of the literature. *Journal of Visual Impairment and Blindness, 85*(2), 58–61.

Esposito, C., Cole, C. L., Shapiro, E. S., & Bambara, L. *Self-management and cognitive tactics for improving study behavior and academic performance among high school biology students*. Manuscript submitted for publication.

Evans, I. M. (1991). Testing and diagnosis: A review and evaluation. In L. H. Meyer, C. A. Peck, & L. Brown (Eds.), *Critical issues in the lives of people with severe disabilities* (pp. 25–44). Baltimore, MD: Paul H. Brookes.

Fantuzzo, J. W., & Polite, K. (1990). School-based, behavioral self-management: A review and analysis. *School Psychology Quarterly 5*, 180–198.

Fantuzzo, J. W., Polite, K., Cook, D. M., & Quinn, G. (1988). An evaluation of the effectiveness of teacher- vs. student-management interventions with elementary school students. *Psychology in the Schools, 25*, 154–163.

Fantuzzo, J. W., Rohrbeck, C. A., & Azar, S. T. (1987). A component analysis of behavioral self-management interventions with elementary school students. *Child & Family Behavior Therapy, 9*(1–2), 33–43.

Feindler, E., Marriott, S., & Iwata, M. (1984). Group anger control training for junior high school dropouts. *Cognitive Therapy and Research, 8*, 299–311.

Feldman, M. P., & Peay, J. (1982). Ethical and legal issues. In A. S. Bellack, M. Hersen, & A. E. Kazdin (Eds.), *International handbook of behavior modification and therapy* (pp. 231–261). New York: Plenum Press.

Fine, S., Gilbert, M., Schmidt, L., & Haley, G. (1989). Short-term group therapy with depressed adolescents. *Canadian Journal of Psychiatry, 34*, 97–102.

Fish, M. C., & Mendola, L. R. (1986). The effect of self-instruction training on homework completion in an elementary special education class. *School Psychology Review, 15*, 268-276.

Fox, D. E., & Kendall, P. C. (1983). Thinking through academic problems: Application of cognitive-behavior therapy to learning. In T. R. Kratochwill (Ed.), *Advances in School Psychology* (Vol. 3, pp. 269–301). Hillsdale, NJ: Erlbaum.

Fremouw, W. J., & Zitter, R. E. (1978). A comparison of skills training and cognitive restructuring relaxation for the treatment of speech anxiety. *Behavior Therapy, 9*, 248–259.

Friedling, C., & O'Leary, S. G. (1979). Effects of self-instructional training on second- and third-grade hyperactive children: A failure to replicate. *Journal of Applied Behavior Analysis, 12*, 211–219.

Gardner, W. I., Clees, T. J., & Cole, C. L. (1983). Self-management of disruptive verbal ruminations by a mentally retarded adult. *Applied Research in Mental Retardation, 4*, 41–58.

Gardner, W. I., & Cole, C. L. (1988). Self-monitoring procedures. In E. S. Shapiro & T. R. Kratochwill (Eds.), *Behavioral assessment in schools* (pp. 206–246). New York: Guilford Press.

Gardner, W. I., Cole, C. L., Berry, D. L., & Nowinski, J. M. (1983). Reduction of disruptive behaviors in mentally retarded adults: A self-management approach. *Behavior Modification, 7*, 76–96.

Gaylord-Ross, R., & Haring, T. (1987). Social interaction research for adolescents with severe handicaps. *Behavioral Disorders, 12*, 264–275.

Giangreco, M. F., & Meyer, L. H. (1988). Expanding service delivery options in regular schools and classrooms for students with severe disabilities. In J. L. Graden, J. E. Zins, & M. J. Curtis (Eds.), *Alternative educational delivery systems: Enhancing instructional options for all students* (pp. 241–267). Washington, DC: National Association of School Psychologists.

Gifford, J. L., Rusch, F. R., Martin, J. E., & White, D. M. (1984). Autonomy and adaptability: A proposed technology for maintaining work behavior. In N. Ellis & N. Bray (Eds.), *International review of research in mental retardation* (Vol. 12, pp. 285–318). New York: Academic Press.

Glomb, N., & West, R. P. (1990). Teaching behaviorally disordered adolescents to use self-management skills for improving the completeness, accuracy, and neatness of creative writing homework assignments. *Behavioral Disorders, 15* 233–242.

Glynn, E. L., & Thomas, J. D. (1974). Effect of cueing on self-control of classroom behavior. *Journal of Applied Behavior Analysis, 7*, 299–306.

Goldstein, A. P., & Pentz, M. A. (1984). Psychological skill training and the aggressive adolescent. *School Psychology Review, 13*, 311–323.

Goldstein, A. P., Sprafkin, R. P., Gershaw, N. J., & Klein, P. (1980). *Skill-streaming the adolescent: A structured learning approach to teaching prosocial skills*. Champaign, IL: Research Press.

Green, C. W., Reid, D. H., White, L. K., Halford, R. C., Brittain, D. P., & Gardner, S. M. (1988). Identifying reinforcers for persons with profound handicaps: Staff opinion versus systematic assessment of preferences. *Journal of Applied Behavior Analysis, 22*, 31–43.

Gresham, F. M. (1985). Utility of cognitive–behavioral procedures for social skills training with children: A critical review. *Journal of Abnormal Child Psychology, 13*, 411–423.

Gresham, F. M., & Elliott, S. N. (1990). *Social Skills Rating System: Manual*. Circle Pines, MN: American Guidance Service.

Grossman, P. B., & Hughes, J. N. (1992). Self-control interventions with internalizing disorders: A review and analysis. *School Psychology Review, 21*, 229–245.

Guess, D., Benson, H. S., & Siegel-Causey, E. (1985). Concepts and issues related to choice-making and autonomy among persons with severe disabilities. *Journal of the Association for Persons with Severe Handicaps, 10*, 79–86.

Guess, D., & Helmstetter, E. (1986). Skill cluster instruction and the individualized curriculum sequencing model. In R. Horner, L. Meyer, & H. D. Fredericks (Eds.), *Education of learners with severe handicaps: Exemplary service strategies* (pp. 221–248). Baltimore: Paul H. Brookes.

Guess, D., Sailor, W., & Baer, D. M. (1976). *Functional speech and language training for the severely handicapped* (Part 2). Lawrence, KS: H & H Enterprises, Inc.

Guess, D., & Siegel-Causey, E. (1985). Behavioral control and education of severely handicapped students: Who's doing what to whom? and why? In D. Bricker & J. Filler (Eds.), *Severe mental retardation: From theory to practice* (pp. 230–244). Reston, VA: The Division of Mental Retardation of the Council for Exceptional Children.

Hallahan, D. P., Lloyd, J. W., Kneedler, R. D., & Marshall, K. J. (1982). A camparison of the effects of self- versus teacher-assessment of on-task behavior. *Behavior Therapy, 12*, 715–723.

Hallahan, D. P., Marshall, K. J., & Lloyd, J. W. (1981). Self-recording during group instruction: Effects on attention to task. *Learning Disability Quarterly, 4*, 407–413.

Hanel, F., & Martin, G. (1980). Self-monitoring, self-administration of token reinforcement, and goal-setting to improve work rates with retarded clients. *International Journal of Rehabilitation Research, 3*, 505–517.

Hansen, D. J., Watson-Perczel, M., & Christopher, J. S. (1989). Clinical issues in social skills training with adolescents. *Clinical Psychology Review, 9*, 365–391.

Hardman, M. L., Drew, C. J., Egan, M. W., & Wolf, B. (1990). *Human exceptionality* (3rd ed.). Boston, MA: Allyn and Bacon.

Harris, K. R. (1986). Self-monitoring of attentional behavior versus self-monitoring of productivity: Effects on on-task behavior and academic response rate among learning disabled children. *Journal of Applied Behavior, 19*, 417–423.

Hazel, J. S., Schumaker, J. B., Sherman, J. A., & Sheldon-Wildgen, J. (1981). *Asset: A social skills program for adolescents.* Champaign, IL: Research Press.

Henning, J., & Dalrymple, N. (1986). A guide for developing social and leisure programs for students with autism. In E. Schopler & G. B. Mesibov (Eds.), *Social behavior in autism* (pp. 321–350). New York: Plenum.

Holman, J., & Baer, D. M. (1979). Facilitating generalization of on-task behavior through self-monitoring of academic tasks. *Journal of Autism and Developmental Disabilities, 9*, 429–446.

Horner, R. H. (1991). The future of applied behavior analysis for people with severe disabilities: Commentary I. In L. H. Meyer, C. A. Peck, & L. Brown (Eds.), *Critical issues in the lives of people with severe disabilities* (pp. 607–611). Baltimore, MD: Paul H. Brookes.

Horner, R. H., Meyer, L. H., & Fredericks, H. D. B. (1986). *Education of learners with severe handicaps: Exemplary service strategies.* Baltimore: Paul H. Brookes.

Houghton, J., Bronicki, G. J. B., & Guess, D. (1987). Opportunities to express preferences and make choices among students with severe disabilities in classroom settings. *Journal of the Association for Persons with Severe Handicaps, 12*, 18–27.

Hughes, C. A., & Boyle, J. R. (1991). Effects of self-monitoring for on-task behavior and task productivity on elementary students with moderate mental retardation. *Education and Treatment of Children. 14*, 96–111.

Hughes, C. A., & Hendrickson, J. M. (1987). Self-monitoring with at-risk students in the regular class setting. *Education and Treatment of Children, 10*, 236–250.

Hughes, C. A., Korinek, L., & Gorman, J. (1991). Self-management for students with mental retardation in public school settings: A research review. *Education and Training in Mental Retardation, 26*, 271–291.

Hughes, C. A., Ruhl, K. L., & Misra, A. (1989). Self-management research with behaviorally disordered students in school settings: A promise unfulfilled? *Behavioral Disorders, 14*, 250–262.

Hughes, J. N., & Sullivan, K. A. (1988). Outcome assessment in social skills training with children. *Journal of School Psychology, 26*, 167–183.

Inderbitzen-Pizaruk, H., & Foster, S. L. (1990). Adolescent friendships and peer acceptance: Implications for social skills training. *Clinical Psychology Review. 10*, 425–439.

Jacobson, E. (1938). *Progressive relaxation.* Chicago: University of Chicago Press.

Johnston, M. B., Whitman, T. L., & Johnson, M. (1980). Teaching addition and subtraction to mentally retarded children: A self-instruction program. *Applied Research in Mental Retardation, 1,* 141–160.

Jason, L., & Burrows, B. (1983). Transition training for high school seniors. *Cognitive Therapy Research, 7,* 79–92.

Kamii, C. (1991). Toward autonomy: The importance of critical thinking and choice making. *School Psychology Review, 20,* 382–388.

Kanfer, F. H. (1977). The many faces of self-control. In R. B. Stuart (Ed.), *Behavioral self-management: Strategies, techniques, and outcomes* (pp. 1–48). New York: Brunner/Mazel.

Kanfer, F. H., & Gaelick, L. (1986). Self-management methods. In F. H. Kanfer & A. P. Goldstein (Eds.), *Helping people change: A textbook of methods* (3rd ed., pp. 283–345). New York: Pergamon Press.

Kapadia, E. S., & Fantuzzo, J. W. (1988). Effects of teacher- and self-administered procedures on the spelling performance of learning-handicapped children. *Journal of School Psychology, 26,* 49–58.

Kazdin, A. E. (1975). *Behavior modification in applied settings.* Homewood, IL: Dorsey Press.

Kehle, T. J., Clark, E., Jenson, W. R., & Wampold, B. E. (1986). Effectiveness of self-observation with behavior disordered elementary school children. *School Psychology Review, 15,* 289–295.

Kendall, P. C., & Braswell, L. (1985). *Cognitive–behavioral therapy for impulsive children.* New York: Guilford Press.

Kendall, P. C., & Finch, A. J. (1978). A cognitive–behavioral treatment for impulsivity: A group comparison study. *Journal of Consulting and Clinical Psychology, 46,* 110–118.

Keogh, B. K., & Hall, R. J. (1984). Cognitive training with learning-disabled pupils. In A. W. Meyers & W. E. Craighead (Eds.), *Cognitive behavior therapy with children* (pp. 163–191). New York: Plenum Press.

Keogh, D. A., Faw, G. D., Whitman, T. L., & Reid, D. H. (1984). Enhancing leisure skills in severely retarded adolescents through a self-instructional treatment package. *Analysis and Intervention in Developmental Disabilities, 4,* 333–351.

Klein, R. D. (1979). Modifying academic performance in the grade school classroom. In M. Hersen, R. M. Eisler, & P. M. Miller (Eds.), *Progress in behavior modification* (Vol. 8, pp. 293–321). New York: Academic Press.

Knapczyk, D. R. (1988). Reducing aggressive behaviors in special and regular class settings by training alternative social responses. *Behavioral Disorders, 14,* 27–39.

Koegel, R. L., Dyer, D., & Bell, L. K. (1987). The influence of child-preferred activities on autistic children's social behavior. *Journal of Applied Behavior Analysis, 20,* 243–252.

Koegel, R. L., & Koegel, L. K. (1989). Community-referenced research on self-stimulation. In E. Cipani, (Ed.), *The treatment of severe behavior disorders: Behavior analysis approaches* (pp. 129–150). Washington, DC: American Association on Mental Retardation.

Kratochwill, T. R., & Morris, R. J. (Eds.). (1991). *The practice of child therapy* (2nd ed.). New York: Pergamon Press.

Lalli, E. P., & Shapiro, E. S. (1990). The effects of self-monitoring and contingent reward on sight word acquisition. *Education and Treatment of Children, 12,* 129–141.

Lam, A. L., Cole, C. L., Shapiro, E. S., & Bambara, L. M. (in press). Relative effects of self-monitoring, on-task behavior, academic accuracy, and disruptive behavior in students with behavior disorders. *School Psychology Review.*

Lazarus, A. A. (1976). *Multi-modal behavior therapy.* New York: Springer.

Lazarus, A. A. (1977). *In the mind's eye.* New York: Rawson Associates.

Lenz, R. K. (1992). Self-managed learning strategy systems for children and youth. *School Psychology Review, 21,* 211–228.

Litrownik, A. J., White, K., McInnis, E. T., & Licht, B. G. (1984). A process of self-management programs for the developmentally disabled. *Analysis and Intervention in Developmental Disabilities, 4,* 189–198.

Lloyd, J. W., Bateman, D. F., Landrum, T. J. & Hallahan, D. P. (1989). Self-recording of attention versus productivity. *Journal of Applied Behavior Analysis, 22,* 315–324.

Lochman, J. E., & Curry, J. F. (1986). Effects of social problem-solving training and self-instruction with aggressive boys. *Journal of Clinical Child Psychology, 15,* 159–164.

Luria, A. R. (1961). *The role of speech in the regulation of normal and abnormal behaviors.* New York: Liverwright.

Mace, F. C., & Kratochwill, T. R. (1985). Theories of reactivity in self-monitoring: A comparison of cognitive–behavioral and operant models. *Behavior Modification, 9,* 323–344.

Mace, F. C., Shapiro, E. S., West, B. J., Campbell, C., & Altman, J. (1986). The role of reinforcement in reactive self-monitoring. *Applied Research in Mental Retardation, 7,* 315–327.

Mace, F. C., & West, B. J. (1986). Unresolved theoretical issues in self-management: Implications for research and practice. *Professional School Psychology, 1,* 149–163.

Mahoney, M. J., & Arnkoff, D. (1978). Cognitive and self-control therapies. In S. L. Garfield & A. E. Bergin (Eds.), *Handbook of psychotherapy and behavior change* (2nd ed., pp. 689–722). New York: Wiley.

Mar, H. H. (1991). Retooling psychology to serve children and adolescents with severe disabilities. *School Psychology Review, 20,* 510–521.

Martens, B. K., & Meller, P. J. (1990). The application of behavioral principles to educational settings. In T. B. Gutkin & C. R. Reynolds (Eds.), *The handbook of school psychology* (2nd ed., pp. 612–634). New York: Wiley.

Martens, B. K., Witt, J. C., Elliott, S. N., & Darveaux, D. (1985). Teacher judgments concerning the acceptability of school based interventions. *Professional Psychology, 16,* 191–198.

Martin, J., Rusch, R., James, V., Decker, P., & Trtol, K. (1982). The use of picture cues to establish self-control in the preparation of complex meals by mentally retarded adults. *Applied Research in Mental Retardation*, *3*, 105–119.

Mash, E. J., & Barkley, R. A. (Eds.). (1989). *Treatment of childhood disorders*. New York: Guilford Press.

McConnell, S. R. (1987). Entrapment effects and the generalization and maintenance of social skills training for elementary school students with behavioral disorders. *Behavioral Disorders, 12,* 252–263.

McCurdy, B. L., & Shapiro, E. S. (1988). Self-observation and the reduction of inappropriate classroom behavior. *Journal of School Psychology, 26,* 371–378.

McEvoy, M. A., & Odom, S. L. (1987). Social interaction training for preschool children with behavioral disorders. *Behavioral Disorders, 12,* 242–251.

McGinnis, E., & Goldstein, A. P. (1984). *Skillstreaming the elementary school child: A guide for teaching prosocial skills*. Champaign, IL: Research Press.

McGinnis, E., & Goldstein, A. P. (1992). *Skillstreaming in early childhood: Teaching prosocial skills to the preschool and kindergarten child*. Champaign, IL: Research Press.

McIntosh, R., Vaughn, S., & Zaragoza, N. (1991). A review of social interventions for students with learning disabilities. *Journal of Learning, 24,* 451–458.

McLaughlin, T. F. (1984). A comparison of self-recording and self-recording plus consequences for on-task and assignment completion. *Contemporary Educational Psychology, 9,* 185–192.

McLaughlin, T. F., Burgess, N., & Sackville-West, L. (1982). Effects of self-recording and self-recording + matching on academic performance. *Child Behavior Therapy, 3*(2–3), 17–27.

McLaughlin, T. F., & Truhlicka, M. (1983). Effects on academic performance of self-recording and matching with behaviorally disordered students: A replication. *Behavioral Engineering, 8,* 69–74.

Meichenbaum, D. H. (1972). Cognition modification of test anxious college students. *Journal of Consulting and Clinical Psychology, 39,* 370–380.

Meichenbaum, D. (1977). *Cognitive–behavior modification*. New York: Plenum Press.

Meichenbaum, D. (1985). *Stress inoculation training*. New York: Pergamon Press.

Meichenbaum, D. H., & Goodman, J. (1971). Training impulsive children to talk to themselves: A means of developing self-control. *Journal of Abnormal Psychology, 77,* 115–126.

Meyer, L. H. (1985). *Program quality indicators: A checklist of the most promising practices in programs for students with severe disabilities*. Syracuse, NY: Syracuse University, Division of Special Education and Rehabilitation.

Meyer, L. H. (1987). *Program quality indicators: A checklist of the most promising practices in educational programs for students with severe disabilities* (rev. ed.).

Syracuse, NY: Syracuse University, Division of Special Education and Rehabilitation.

Meyer, L. H., Peck, C. A., & Brown, L. (Eds.). (1991). *Critical issues in the lives of people with severe disabilities*. Baltimore, MD: Paul H. Brookes.

Miller, L. H., Hale, G. A., & Stevenson, H. W. (1968). Learning and problem solving by retarded and normal Ss. *American Journal of Mental Deficiency, 72,* 681–690.

Miller, M., Miller, S. R., Wheeler, J. J. & Selinger, J. (1989). Can a single-classroom treatment approach change academic performance and behavioral characteristics in severely behaviorally disordered adolescents: An experimental inquiry. *Behavioral Disorders, 14,* 215–225.

Minner, S. (1990). Use of a self-recording procedure to decrease the time taken by behaviorally disordered students to walk to special classes. *Behavioral Disorders, 15,* 210–216.

Mithaug, D. E., & Hanawalt, D. A. (1978). The validation of procedures to assess prevocational task preferences in retarded adults. *Journal of Applied Behavior Analysis, 11,* 153–162.

Mithaug, D. E., & Mar, D. K. (1980). The relation between choosing and working prevocational tasks in two severely retarded young adults. *Journal of Applied Behavior Analysis, 13,* 177–182.

Moore, L. A., Waguespack, A. M., Wickstrom, K. F., Witt, J. C., & Gaydos, G. R. (in press). Mystery motivator: An effective and time effecient intervention. *School Psychology Review.*

Morrow, L. W., & Presswood, S. (1984). The effects of self-control techniques on eliminating three stereotypic behaviors in a multiple-handicapped institutionalized adolescent. *Behavioral Disorders, 9,* 247–253.

Musante, L., Gilbert, M. A., & Thibaut, J. (1983). The effects of control in perceived fairness of procedures and outcomes. *Journal of Experimental Social Psychology, 19,* 223–238.

Nagel, D. A., Schumaker, J. B., & Deshler, D. D. (1986). *The learning strategies curriculum: The first-letter mnemonic strategy.* Lawrence, KS: The University of Kansas.

Narayan, J. S., Heward, W. L., Gardner, R., Courson, F. H., & Omness, C. K. (1990). Using response cards to increase student participation in an elementary classroom. *Journal of Applied Behavior Analysis, 21,* 483–490.

Nelson, J. R., Smith, D. J., Young, R. K., & Dodd, J. (1991). A review of self-management outcome research conducted with students who exhibit behavioral disorders. *Behavioral Disorders, 16,* 169–179.

Nelson, R. O. (1977). Assessment and therapeutic functions of self-monitoring. In M. Hersen, R. M. Eisler, & P. M. Miller (Eds.), *Progress in behavior modification* (Vol. 5, pp. 263–308). New York: Academic Press.

Novaco, R. W. (1977a). Stress inoculation: A cognitive therapy for anger and its application to a case of depression. *Journal of Consulting and Clinical Psychology, 45,* 600–608.

Novaco, R. W. (1977b). A stress inoculation approach to anger management in the training of law enforcement officers. *American Journal of Community Psychology, 5*, 327–346.

Novaco, R. W. (1978). Anger and coping with stress. In J. P. Foreyt & D. P. Rathjen (Eds.), *Cognitive behavior therapy: Research and application* (pp. 135–173). New York: Plenum Press.

Parsons, M. B., & Reid, D. H. (1990). Assessing food preferences among persons with profound mental retardation: Providing opportunities to make choices. *Journal of Applied Behavior Analysis, 23*, 183–195.

Parsons, M. B., Reid, D. H., Reynolds, J., & Bumgarner, M. (1990). Effects of chosen versus assigned jobs on the work performance of persons with severe handicaps. *Journal of Applied Behavior Analysis, 23*, 253–258.

Peck, C. A. (1991). Linking values and science in social policy decisions affecting citizens with severe disabilities. In L. H. Meyer, C. A. Peck, & L. Brown (Eds.), *Critical issues in the lives of people with severe disabilities* (pp. 1–15). Baltimore, MD: Paul H. Brookes.

Peterson, L., & Shigetomi, C. (1981). The use of coping techniques to minimize anxiety in hospitalized children. *Behavior Therapy, 12*, 1–14.

Piersel, W. C. (1985). Self-observation and completion of school assignments: The influence of a physical recording device and expectancy characteristics. *Psychology in the Schools, 22*, 331–336.

Pigott, H. E., Fantuzzo, J. W., Heggie, D. L., & Clement, P. W. (1985). A student-administered group-oriented contingency intervention: Its efficacy in a regular classroom. *Child & Family Behavior Therapy, 6*, 41–55.

Prater, M. A., Joy, R., Chilman, B., Temple, J., & Miller, S. R. (1991). Self-monitoring of on-task behavior by adolescents with learning disabilities. *Learning Disability Quarterly, 14*. 164–178.

Reese, R. M. (1986). *Teaching individual and group problem solving to adults with mental retardation.* Unpublished doctoral dissertation, University of Kansas, Lawrence.

Reid, D. H., & Parsons, M. B. (1991). Making choice a routine part of mealtimes for persons with profound mental retardation. *Behavioral Residential Treatment, 6*, 249–261.

Rhode, G., Jenson, W. R., & Reavis, H. K. (1992). *The tough kid book.* Longmont, CO: Sopriswest, Inc.

Rhode, G., Morgan, D. P. & Young, K. R. (1983). Generalization and maintenance of treatment gains of behaviorally handicapped students from resource rooms to regular classrooms using self-evaluation procedures. *Journal of Applied Behavior Analysis, 16*, 171–188.

Rice, M. S., & Nelson, D. L. (1988). Effect of choice making on a self-care activity in mentally retarded adult and adolescent males. *The Occupational Therapy Journal of Research, 8*, 176–185.

Richter, F. D., & Tjosvold, D. (1980). Effects of student participation in classroom decision making on attitudes, peer interaction, motivation, and learning. *Journal of Applied Psychology, 65*, 74–80.

Roberts, R. N., & Dick, M. L. (1982). Self-control in the classroom: Theoretical issues and practical applications. In T. R. Kratochwill (Ed.), *Advances in School Psychology* (Vol. 2, pp. 275–314). Hillsdale, NJ: Lawrence Erlbaum.

Roberts, R. N., Nelson, R. O., & Olson, T. W. (1987). Self-instruction: An analysis of the differential effects of instruction and reinforcement. *Journal of Applied Behavior Analysis, 20,* 235–242.

Robertson, S. J., Simon, S. J., Pachman, J. S., & Drabman, R. S. (1979). Self-control and generalization procedures in a classroom of disruptive retarded children. *Child Behavior Therapy, 1,* 347–362.

Robinson-Wilson, A. (1977). Picture recipe cards as an approach to teaching severely and profoundly retarded adults to cook. *Education and Training of the Mentally Retarded, 12,* 69–73.

Rudrud, E. H., Rice, J. M., Robertson, J. M., & Olson, N. M. (1984). The use of self-monitoring to increase and maintain production rates. *Vocational Evaluation and Work Adjustment Bulletin, 17,* 14–17.

Safran, J. D., Alden, L. E., & Davidson, P. O. (1980). Client anxiety level as a moderator variable in assertion training. *Cognitive Therapy and Research, 4,* 189–200.

Schneider, B. H. (1992). Didactic methods for enhancing children's peer relations: A quantitative review. *Clinical Psychology Review, 12,* 363–382.

Schumaker, J. B., Deshler, D. D., Alley, G. R., Warner, M. M., Clark, F. L., & Nolan, S. (1982). Error monitoring: A learning strategy for improving adolescents' academic performance. In W. M. Cruickshank & J. W. Lerner (Eds.), *Coming of age: Vol. 3 The Best of ACLD* (pp. 170–183). Syracuse, NY: Syracuse University Press.

Schumaker, J. B., Deshler, D. D., Alley, G. R., Warner, M. M., & Denton, P. H. (1982). Multipass: A learning strategy for improving reading comprehension. *Learning Disability Quarterly, 5,* 295–304.

Shapiro, E. S. (1981). Self-control procedures with the mentally retarded. In M. Hersen, R. M. Eisler, & P. M. Miller (Eds.), *Progress in behavior modification* (Vol. 12, pp. 265–297). New York: Academic Press.

Shapiro, E. S. (1989a). Teaching self-management skills to learning disabled adolescents. *Learning Disability Quarterly, 12,* 275–287.

Shapiro, E. S. (1989b). *Academic skills problems: Direct assessment and intervention.* New York: Guilford Press.

Shapiro, E. S., & Ackerman, A. (1983). Increasing productivity rates in adult mentally retarded clients: The failure of self-monitoring. *Applied Research Mental Retardation, 4,* 163–181.

Shapiro, E. S., Albright, T. S., & Ager, C. L. (1986). Group versus individual contingencies in modifying two disruptive adolescents' behavior. *Professional School Psychology, 1,* 105–116.

Shapiro, E. S., Browder, D. M., & D'Huyvetters, K. K. (1984). Increasing academic productivity of severely multihandicapped children with self-management: Idiosyncratic effects. *Analysis and Intervention in Developmental Disabilities, 4,* 171–188.

Shapiro, E. S., & Cole, C. L. (1992). Self-monitoring. In T. H. Ollendick &

M. Hersen (Eds.), *Handbook of child and adolescent assessment* (pp. 124–139). New York: Pergamon Press.

Shapiro, E. S., McGonigle, J. J., & Ollendick, T. H. (1981). An analysis of self-assessment and self-reinforcement in a self-managed token economy with mentally retarded children. *Applied Research in Mental Retardation, 1,* 227–240.

Shapiro, E. S., & McQuillan, K. (1986). *Self-management for LD adolescents: A training program.* Unpublished manuscript, Lehigh University, Bethlehem, PA.

Shear, S. M., & Shapiro, E. S. (in press). The effects of using self-recording and self-observation in reducing disruptive behavior. *Journal of School Psychology.*

Shevin, M., & Klein, N. K. (1984). The importance of choice-making skills for students with severe disabilities. *Journal of the Association for Persons with Severe Handicaps, 9,* 159–166.

Shores, R. E. (1987). Overview of research on social interaction: A historical and personal perspective. *Behavioral Disorders, 12,* 233–241.

Shure, M. B. (1992a). *I can problem solve: An interpersonal cognitive problem-solving program (intermediate elementary grades).* Champaign, IL: Research Press.

Shure, M. B. (1992b). *I can problem solve: An interpersonal cognitive problem-solving program (kindergarten & primary grades).* Champaign, IL: Research Press.

Shure, M. B. (1992c). *I can problem solve: An interpersonal cognitive problem-solvinig program (preschool).* Champaign, IL: Research Press.

Siegel, L. J., & Peterson, L. (1980). Stress reduction in young dental patients through coping skills and sensory information. *Journal of Consulting and Clinical Psychology, 48,* 785–787.

Sigafoos, J., & Dempsey, R. (1992). Assessing choice making among children with multiple disabilities. *Journal of Applied Behavior Analysis, 25,* 747–755.

Singh, N. N., Deitz, D. E., Epstein, M. H. & Singh, J. (1991). Social behavior of students who are seriously emotionally disturbed: A quantitative analysis of intervention studies. *Behavior Modification, 15,* 74–94.

Skinner, C. H., Turco, T., Beatty, K., & Rasavage, C. (1989). Cover, copy, and compare: A method for increasing multiplication performance. *School Psychology Review, 18,* 412–420.

Smith, D. J., Young, K. R., Nelson, J. R. & West, R. P. (1992). The effect of a self-management procedure on the classroom academic behavior of students with mild handicaps. *School Psychology Review, 21,* 59–72.

Smith, D. J., Young, R., West, R. P., Morgan, D. P., & Rhode, G. (1988). Reducing the disruptive behavior of junior high school students: A classroom self-management procedure. *Behavioral Disorders, 13,* 231–239.

Snider, V. E. (1987). Use of self-monitoring of attention with LD students: Research and application. *Learning Disabilities Quarterly, 10*(2), 139–151.

Spivack, G., & Shure, M. G. (1974). *Social adjustment of young children: A cognitive approach to solving real-life problems.* San Francisco: Jossey-Bass.

Spivack, G., Platt, J. J., & Shure, M. B. (1976). *The problem-solving approach to adjustment.* San Francisco: Jossey-Bass.

Stern, J. B. & Fodor, I. G. (1989). Anger control in children: A review of social skills and cognitive–behavioral approaches to dealing with aggressive children. *Child and Family Behavior Therapy, 11*(3–4), 1–20.

Stevens, K. B., Blackhurst, A. E., & Slaton, D. B. (1991). Teaching memorized spelling with a microcomputer: Time delay and computer-assisted instruction. *Journal of Applied Behavior Analysis, 24,* 153–160.

Stokes, T. F. & Baer, D. M. (1977). An implicit technology of generalization. *Journal of Applied Behavior Analysis, 10,* 349–367.

Stokes, T. F., & Osnes, P. G. (1986). Programming the generalization of children's social behavior. In P. S. Strain, M. J. Guralnick, & H. M. Walker (Eds.), *Children's social behavior* (pp. 407–443). Orlando, FL: Academic Press.

Stowitschek, J. J., Ghezzi, P. M., & Safely, K. N. (1987). "I'd rather do it myself": Self-evaluation and correction of handwriting. *Education and Treatment of Children, 10,* 209–224.

Strein, W. (1987). Needs versus deeds: The unfulfilled research potential in school psychology. *Journal of School Psychology, 25,* 3–14.

Swanson, H. L., & Scarpati, S. (1985). Self-instruction training to increase academic performance of educationally handicapped children. *Child and Family Behavior Therapy, 6*(4), 23–39.

Szykula, S. A., Saudargas, R. A., & Wahler, R. G. (1981). The generality of self-control procedures following a change in the classroom teacher. *Education and Treatment of Children, 4,* 253–263.

Tisdelle, D. A. & St. Lawrence, J. S. (1986). Interpersonal problem-solving competency: A review. *Clinical Psychology Review, 6,* 337–356.

Vygotsky, L. (1962). *Thought and language.* New York: Wiley.

Wacker, D., & Berg, W. K. (1983). Effects of picture prompts on the acquisition of complex vocational tasks by mentally retarded adolescents. *Journal of Applied Behavior Analysis, 16,* 417–43.

Wacker, D., & Berg, W. K. (1984). Training adolescents with severe handicaps to set up job tasks independently using picture prompts. *Analysis and Intervention in Developmental Disabilities, 4,* 353–365.

Wacker, D., & Berg, W. K. (1986). Generalizing and maintaining work behavior. In F. R. Rusch (Ed.), *Competitive employment issues and strategies* (pp. 129–140). Baltimore: Paul H. Brookes.

Wasik, B. (1984). *Teaching parents effective problem-solving: A handbook for professionals.* Unpublished manuscript, University of North Carolina, Chapel Hill.

Whalen, C. K., Henker, B., & Hinshaw, S. P. (1985). Cognitive–behavioral therapies for hyperactive children: Premises, problems, and prospects. *Journal of Abnormal Child Psychology, 13,* 391–410.

Whitman, T., & Johnston, M. B. (1983). Teaching addition and subtraction with regrouping to educable mentally retarded children: A group self-instructional program. *Behavior Therapy, 14,* 127–143.

Williams, W., Vogelsberg, R. T., & Schutz, R. P. (1985). Programs for secondary-age severely handicapped youth. In D. Bricker, & J. Filler, (Eds.), *Severe mental retardation: From theory to practice* (pp. 97–118). Lancaster, PA: Division on Mental Retardation of the Council for Exceptional Children.

Wilson, G. T. (1978). Cognitive behavior therapy: Paradigm shift or passing phase? In J. P. Foreyt & D. P. Rathjen (Eds.), *Cognitive behavior therapy: Research and application* (pp. 7–32). New York: Plenum Press.

Witt, J. C. (1986). Teachers' resistance to the use of school-based interventions. *Journal of School Psychology, 24,* 37–44.

Witt, J. C., Moe, G., Gutkin, T. B., & Andrews, L. (1984). The effect of saying the same thing in different ways: The problem of language and jargon in school-based consultation. *Journal of School Psychology, 22,* 361–367.

Wuerch, B., & Voeltz, L. (1982). *Longitudinal leisure skills for severely handicapped learners.* Baltimore: Paul H. Brookes.

Young, K. R., Smith, D. J., West, R. P., & Morgan, D. P. (1987). A peer-mediated program for teaching self-management strategies to adolescents. *Programming for Adolescents with Behavioral Disorders, 3,* 34–47.

Zahavi, A., & Asher, S. R. (1978). The effect of verbal instructions on preschool children's aggressive behavior. *Journal of School Psychology, 16,* 146–153.

Zaragoza, N., Vaughn, S., & McIntosh, R. (1991). Social skills interventions and children with behavior problems: A review. *Behavioral Disorders, 16,* 260–275.

Zeph, L. (1984, November). *The model of C.H.O.I.C.E.: A curriculum framework for incorporating choice making into programs serving students with severe handicaps.* Paper presented at the Eleventh Annual Conference of the Association for Persons with Severe Handicaps, Chicago, IL.

Index